HOW TO BOOST YOUR IN

THERESA CHEUNG is the
and popular psychology bo
Glycaemic Factor: How to I
Sugar. She also co-authored th
Diet Book and has contributed features to *Here's
Health, Health Plus, NHS Mother and Baby, You
Are What You Eat, Red, She* and *Prima* magazines.

Overcoming Common Problems Series

Selected titles

A full list of titles is available from Sheldon Press,
36 Causton Street, London SW1P 4ST and on our website at
www.sheldonpress.co.uk

Introduction

Your invisible bodyguard

Out of sight and out of mind, your immune system is quietly and constantly patrolling your body to detect and destroy invaders. It operates much like an invisible army, mobilizing troops of white blood cells and dispatching them to strategic points around the body where they are on stand-by to fight any invader, be it a virus, a bacterium or a fungus. It's an incredibly complex, sophisticated and effective system, working tirelessly around the clock to protect you and keep you healthy and happy.

A vigorous immune system is vital to good health, both physical and mental. Chronic fatigue, endless colds, allergies, depression, premature ageing and even cancer are some of the all too common manifestations of a weakened immune system, while there is increasing awareness of autoimmune disorders such as rheumatoid arthritis, type 1 diabetes, Sjögren's syndrome, and lupus, in which the immune system attacks the body. The danger is very real. Thousands of people die every year in the UK from influenza, pneumonia and severe sepsis. Tuberculosis, once considered under control, now also kills thousands of people every year. At the same time, new infectious diseases are emerging around the globe in such forms as severe acute respiratory syndrome (SARS), not to mention the not yet fully understood threat of bird flu.

In response to such threats, the human body has a co-ordinated immune response that is both a marvel of elegant simplicity and an amazingly complex set of biochemical interactions. Usually, your immune system is very effective in warding off disease, but sometimes things go wrong. A bacterium, virus or other microbe might get past your immune defences and make you sick.

Learning how the immune system functions and why things sometimes go wrong is crucial to preventing disease and maximizing your chances of good health. This book takes you on a guided tour through your immune system. Can you boost immunity? Will certain foods and supplements help you fend off infection and disease? Are vaccines necessary? This book sets the record straight by correcting

1

misinformation and giving you all the advice you need to take practical steps to strengthen and support your immune system.

Since we depend so much on our immune system to protect us from a whole host of hostile invaders, learning how to support and protect our immune system is the most important thing we can do for our health. So, be good to yourself. Read on to discover how to stay free from disease and maximize your potential for high level health and vitality.

1

How your immune system works

Despite its low-key profile, the immune system is the subject of great attention both in the laboratories of prominent scientists and on the shelves of shops carrying countless products that purport to boost or support immunity. Yet most of us know very little about the immune system, how it works, what weakens it and how to strengthen it.

This chapter gives a quick overview of the basic processes involved in order to help you to grasp how the immune system works. Once you understand the basic processes at work, you will be in a much stronger position to understand how certain factors can attack your body's inbuilt defences and how other factors can support them.

What is the immune system?

Your immune system is your basic defence against poor health. It fights a secret war against the constant invasions and attacks made on your body by micro-organisms in the environment. If your immune defences are working at their optimum level of efficiency you are unlikely to notice any symptoms. If, however, you feel you are constantly unwell, permanently tired or just below par, this could suggest that your immune defences are not doing their job effectively.

A healthy, properly functioning immune system is absolutely vital to good health. It is the key to the healing process, from the tiniest scratch to the most complex virus. Even the ageing process is intimately linked with the immune system. Compromised immunity leaves us vulnerable to disease and impairs our ability to heal properly and to age well.

How does the immune system work?

Your immune system is made up of a network of cells, tissues and organs that work together to protect your body. Through a vital series of steps called the immune response it has the essential job of neutralizing or destroying any invading micro-organisms so that you stay disease-free.

The cells that form a crucial part of this defence system are called white blood cells or leucocytes. Leucocytes are produced or stored in many locations throughout the body, including the thymus, the spleen and the bone marrow, which are called the lymphoid organs. There are also clumps of lymphoid tissue throughout the body, primarily in the form of lymph nodes that house the leucocytes.

The leucocytes circulate through the body between the organs and lymph nodes by means of the lymphatic vessels. Leucocytes can also circulate through the blood vessels. In this way, the immune system works in a co-ordinated manner to monitor the body for substances that might cause problems.

Leucocytes come in two basic types – phagocytes and lymphocytes, which combine to seek out and destroy the organisms or substances that cause disease.

Phagocytes are cells that chew up invading organisms. The most common type of phagocyte is the neutrophil, whose job is to fight bacteria. So when doctors are worried about a bacterial infection, sometimes they order a blood test to see if a patient has an increased number of neutrophils triggered by the infection. Other types of phagocytes have their own job to make sure that the body responds appropriately to a specific type of invader.

Lymphocytes are cells that allow the body to remember and recognize previous invaders. There are two kinds of lymphocytes: B lymphocytes and T lymphocytes (also often known simply as B cells and T cells). Lymphocytes start out in the bone marrow and either mature there into B cells or leave for the thymus gland, where they mature into T cells. B lymphocytes and T lymphocytes have separate jobs to do: B lymphocytes are like the body's military intelligence system, seeking out their targets and sending defences to locate them. T cells are like the soldiers, destroying the invaders that the intelligence system has identified.

A crucial part of the immune system is the lymphatic system, which produces immune cells and provides transport for them. The lymphatic system is composed of a network of lymphatic vessels that transport a fluid derived from blood called lymph fluid or simply lymph. Lymph, a transparent yellowish fluid, bathes the body's tissues with white blood cells, fighting cancer, viruses, bacteria, and infections. Every 24 hours, approximately 5 gallons (about 23 litres) of lymph pass from the bloodstream to body tissues, providing oxygen and nutrients to cells and carrying away toxins and by-products.

In addition to the lymphatic vessels, the lymphatic system also includes lymphoid organs in which the lymphocytes (see above) are produced. Lymph nodes, also called lymph glands, are small pea-shaped structures that are most obvious in the neck, under the arms and in the groin, but they are found throughout the body. Their function is to serve as meeting places for cells of the immune system. The immune cells travel to these nodes via lymph ducts, and when your body is fighting an unusually strong pathogen or group of pathogens, your lymph nodes fill with immune cells and become swollen and tender to the touch. (A pathogen is any disease-causing agent, for example, some types of viruses and bacteria.) This is why doctors examine lymph glands when they suspect cancer or other powerful illnesses.

Immunity in three acts

We have three types of immunity – passive, innate, and adaptive.

Passive immunity

Passive immunity is 'borrowed' from another source and it lasts for a short time. For example, antibodies in a mother's breast milk provide an infant with temporary immunity to diseases that the mother has been exposed to. This can help to protect the infant against infection during the early years of childhood and is essential protection while babies are developing their own immune system.

Innate immunity

Everyone is born with innate (or natural) immunity, a type of general protection that all humans have. The innate immune response is similar to your local police force and is always available to jump in and eliminate or contain an infection. An important part of your 'local police force' are the neutrophils, specialized cells that constantly patrol the bloodstream looking for trouble. If they get a signal from a tissue that there might be danger they immediately leave the blood vessel and go into the tissue and try to engulf and kill any enemies they encounter.

Innate immunity also includes the external barriers of the body, like the skin and mucous membranes (i.e. the membranes that line the nose, throat and gastrointestinal tract), which are our first line of defence in preventing diseases from entering the body. Skin has a vitally important protective role to play in our health. This essential covering is designed to keep things in (such as blood, organs, bones, muscles) and to keep us in shape, but it also keeps unwelcome visitors out. Any break in skin can lead to infection, and if this outer defence is broken (as happens when you get a cut or bruise) the skin attempts to heal the cut quickly, and special immune cells on the skin attack invading germs. Given this crucial function, skin needs to be protected and kept as subtle and resilient as possible to keep the chance of infection at bay.

Adaptive immunity

We also have another kind of protection called adaptive (or acquired) immunity. This type of immunity develops throughout our lives in response to contact with any new bacteria or viruses or when we are immunized against disease through vaccination. Once immunity has developed in response to these micro-organisms it remains in the memory of the immune system so that if we encounter the same micro-organism in the future, an aggressive response can be put into action very quickly.

While the innate response is working on the local front lines, the adaptive response system is being marshalled to bring on the full force of your immune militia and find a defence specifically tailored to deal with the pathogen. Typically the adaptive response takes about 5–7 days to get completely mobilized once a pathogen has been detected, and if you have a pathogen that works faster than that, you're in trouble.

The ability to recognize and eliminate foreign invaders is one of the immune system's most impressive attributes, since it allows for the switching on of a series of defence mechanisms in a very short space of time. Although the immune system is capable of diversifying its approach so that it can attack a huge variety of invading organisms, it is important to point out that each micro-organism requires an individualized response. So, for example, if we acquire immunity towards the chickenpox virus, we shall need to develop another immune response to the measles virus if we come into contact with it.

Your immune system in action

When the immune system swings into action against an invader, also called an antigen, the first response comes from the neutrophils, which immediately cluster around areas of trouble in an attempt to kill the enemy. Meanwhile the thymus gland produces T cells, which act together with the B cells produced by the bone marrow. The B cells then produce antibodies to eliminate threatening organisms at the prompting of the T cells. Antibodies are specialized proteins that lock onto specific antigens.

Once the B lymphocytes have produced antibodies, these antibodies continue to exist in a person's body. That means if the same antigen is presented to the immune system again, the antibodies are already there to do their job. That's why if someone gets sick with a certain disease, like chickenpox, that person typically doesn't get sick from it again. This is also why we use immunizations to prevent getting certain diseases. The immunization introduces the body to the antigen in a way that doesn't make a person sick but that does allow the body to produce antibodies that will then protect that person from future attack by the germ or substance that produces that particular disease.

Although antibodies can recognize an antigen and lock onto it, they are not capable of destroying it without help. That is the job of the T cells. The T cells are part of the system that destroys antigens that have been tagged by antibodies or cells that have been infected or somehow changed. (There are actually T cells that are called 'killer cells'.) T cells are also involved in helping signal to other cells (such as phagocytes) to do their jobs.

Antibodies can also neutralize toxins (poisonous or damaging substances) produced by various organisms. Lastly, antibodies can activate a group of proteins called complement, which are also part of the immune system. Complement assists in killing bacteria, viruses or infected cells.

All of these specialized cells and parts of the immune system offer the body protection against disease, and this protection is called immunity. A swift response can be mounted against organisms recognized from the past, but antibody production may take a few days longer if the invading micro organism is new. This is the time when swollen, painful glands can appear, caused by white blood cells incubating a supply of antibodies in the lymph nodes. (The main lymph nodes are found in the armpits, groin and neck.)

What happens to immunity when we age?

Everyone's immune system is different. Some people never seem to get infections, whereas others seem to be ill all the time. As a child gets older, he or she usually becomes immune to more germs as the immune system comes into contact with more and more of them. That's why in general young adults tend to get fewer colds than children – their bodies have learned to recognize many of the viruses that cause colds and can attack them immediately.

Even though our bodies do get more resilient as we leave childhood behind, they also produce fewer T cells as we age, and this means that the ability to fight infection can decline in later life. However, it's encouraging to know that there are things we can do to strengthen our immune system against invaders and to tip the balance towards health. For example, as you'll discover later in the self-defence action plan, good nutrition and regular exercise is vital.[1]

2

Understanding the germs that cause infection

This chapter takes a look at the invaders that your immune system tries to protect you against. Bacteria, viruses and other infectious organisms live everywhere. You can find them in the air; on food, plants and animals; in the soil and in the water; and on just about every other surface – including your own body. They range in size from microscopic single-cell organisms to parasitic worms that can grow to several feet in length. Most of these organisms (or microorganisms, or microbes) won't harm you. But others can cause infection and make you ill.

Your immune system protects you against an abundance of these infectious agents, and at times it's a hard task. Viruses and bacteria are constantly evolving adversaries that are always seeking new ways to attack and defeat your immune system's defences. Here's what your immune system is up against.

Bacteria

Bacteria are one-celled rod- or spiral-shaped organisms that are visible only with a microscope. They're usually self-sufficient and multiply by subdivision. Among the earliest forms of life on earth, bacteria have evolved to survive in a variety of environments. Some can withstand intense heat or cold, and others can survive radiation levels that would be lethal to a human being. Many bacteria, however, prefer the warm and mild environment of a healthy body. Not all bacteria are harmful. In fact, less than 1 per cent cause disease, and some bacteria that live in your body are actually good for you. For instance, *Lactobacillus acidophilus*, a harmless bacterium that resides in your intestines, helps you to digest food, destroys some disease-causing organisms and provides nutrients to your body.

But when harmful infectious bacteria enters your body they can make you ill by rapidly reproducing and producing powerful chemicals that damage cells in the tissue they've invaded. The organism that causes gonorrhoea is an example of a bacterial invader. Others include strains of the bacterium *Escherichia coli*, better known as *E. coli* and often linked to undercooked ground beef, which causes severe gastrointestinal illness. Other conditions caused by bacteria include strep throat and staph infections.

Viruses

A virus is a capsule that contains genetic material – DNA or RNA. Viruses are even tinier than bacteria and can only be seen through electron microscopes, high-powered instruments that produce enlarged images of minute objects. The main mission of a virus is to reproduce. However, unlike bacteria, viruses aren't self-sufficient; they need a suitable host to reproduce. When a virus invades your body, it enters some of your cells and takes over, instructing these host cells to manufacture what it needs for reproduction. Host cells are eventually destroyed during this process.

For example, the influenza virus takes over healthy cells, spreads through your body and causes illness. Signs and symptoms of influenza include fever, chills, muscle aches and malaise. Polio, acquired immunodeficiency syndrome (AIDS) and the common cold are other examples of viral illnesses.

Fungi

Fungi live in the air, in water, in soil and on plants. They can live in your body, and don't always cause illness. Moulds, yeasts and mushrooms are types of fungi. For the most part, these single-celled organisms are slightly larger than bacteria, although some mushrooms are multicellular and plainly visible to the eye – for instance, the mushrooms you may see growing in a wooded area or even in your backyard. Mushrooms aren't infectious, but certain yeasts and moulds can be.

Some fungi are beneficial. For example, penicillin, an antibiotic that kills harmful bacteria in your body, is derived from fungi. Fungi are also essential in making certain foods, such as bread, cheese and yoghurt. Other fungi aren't as beneficial and can cause illness. One example is *Candida*, a yeast infection that can cause vaginal yeast infections and oral thrush.

Protozoa

Protozoa are single-celled organisms that hunt and gather other microbes for food. They can live within your body as a parasite. Many protozoa inhabit your intestinal tract and are harmless, but others cause disease, such as occurred in the 1993 invasion of the Milwaukee water supply by *Cryptosporidium parvum*, which caused thousands of people to become ill. Often, these organisms spend part of their life cycle outside humans or other hosts, living in food, soil, water or insects.

Most protozoa are microscopic, but a minority can grow to an inch or two in diameter. Some protozoa invade your body through the food you eat or the water you drink. Others can be transmitted through sexual contact. Still others are vector-borne, meaning that they rely on another organism to transmit them from person to person. Malaria is an example of a disease caused by a vector-borne protozoan parasite. Mosquitoes are the vector that transmits the deadly parasite *Plasmodium*, which causes the disease.

Helminths

Helminths are larger parasites that can enter your body and take up residence in your intestinal tract, lungs, liver, skin or brain, where they live off the nutrients in your body. The most common helminths are tapeworms and roundworms. Roundworms range in length from about 15cm to 36cm (6 inches to 14 inches) and tapeworms can grow to be 7.5m (about 25 feet) or longer. Tapeworms are made up of hundreds of segments, each of which is capable of breaking off and developing into a new tapeworm.

Understanding infection versus disease

There's a difference between infection and disease. Infection is the first step to disease when bacteria, viruses, or other microbes listed above enter your body and begin to multiply. Disease occurs when the cells in your body are damaged as a result of the infection, and signs and symptoms of illness appear.

It is in response to infection that your immune system springs into action. As we've seen an army of white blood cells (or leucocytes), antibodies and other mechanisms go to war against the microscopic invaders that are causing the infection. For instance, in fighting off the common cold, your body might react with fever, sweats, coughing and sneezing. These are all signs that your immune system is hard at work doing what it does best: fighting for your health.

Usually, your immune system is very effective in warding off infection. But sometimes things go wrong. A bacterium, virus, or

11

other microscopic invader (see Chapter 1) might make it past your immune defences and makes you sick, most typically with a cold or flu.

The common cold

Common cold infections are so widespread that there can be very few people who escape the infection each year. It's called the common cold for good reason, since you are likely to have more colds than any other type of illness.

Over 200 viruses can cause a cold. It has been estimated that adults suffer between two and five colds a year. Children average between three and eight colds a year. They continue getting them throughout childhood. Parents often get them from their children. It's one of the most common reasons that children miss school and parents miss work.

The common cold generally involves a runny nose, nasal congestion and sneezing. You may also have a sore throat, cough, headache, mild fever or other symptoms. Colds can occur year-round, but they occur mostly in the winter (even in areas with mild winters). In areas where there is no winter, colds are most common during the rainy season. When someone has a cold, his or her runny nose is teeming with cold viruses. Sneezing, nose-blowing and nose-wiping spread the virus. You can catch a cold by inhaling the virus if you are sitting close to someone who sneezes, or by touching your nose, eyes or mouth after you have touched something contaminated by the virus. People are most contagious for the first 2–3 days of a cold and usually not contagious at all by 7–10 days.

Once you have 'caught' a cold, the symptoms usually begin in 2 or 3 days, though it may take a week. Typically, an irritated nose or scratchy throat is the first sign, followed within hours by sneezing and a watery nasal discharge. Within 1–3 days, the nasal secretions usually become thicker and perhaps yellow or green. This is a normal part of the common cold and not a reason for antibiotics.

Depending on which virus is the culprit, the virus might also produce other symptoms such as a sore throat, cough, muscle aches, headache and loss of appetite. The entire cold is usually over all by itself in about 7 days, with perhaps a few lingering symptoms (such as cough) for another week. If it lasts longer, consider another problem, such as a sinus infection or allergies.

If you get a cold, over-the-counter cold remedies won't cure it but can relieve your symptoms. It's also important to rest and drink plenty of fluids. Antibiotics should not be used to treat a common cold. They will not help and may make the situation worse! Thick yellow or green nasal discharge is not a reason for antibiotics, unless it lasts for 10–14 days without improving. (In this case, it may be sinusitis.) New antiviral drugs could make runny noses completely clear up a day sooner than usual (and begin to ease the symptoms within a day) but it's unclear whether the benefits of these drugs outweigh the risks. (For information about self-help remedies see Chapter 12.)

Bird flu

Bird flu – known technically as avian influenza – is a highly contagious viral disease affecting mostly chickens, ducks, turkeys, quails and other birds. It was first identified more than 100 years ago. It can be caused by any one of about 20 different strains of the influenza virus. The recent outbreaks in Asia, Turkey and Europe, however, have been largely caused by a highly contagious and virulent strain of the influenza virus known as H5N1. (The name H5N1 refers to the specific nature of two proteins, haemagglutinin and neuraminidase, found on the surface of the virus.)

At present, H5N1 is only slightly infectious to humans who have been in contact with infected birds, and it cannot yet be transmitted from one human to another. However, experts fear that H5N1 may evolve into a virus that can be easily transferred among humans. This, they say, could lead to the first flu pandemic of the 21st century.

According to the US Centers for Disease Control and Prevention, the three great flu pandemics of the 20th century were the result of genetic material from bird flu viruses becoming incorporated into human flu viruses. This led to a far more dangerous virus, which was able to spread rapidly worldwide.

There are two ways in which H5N1 could become a greater threat to human health. One is that the genetic material of the virus could evolve, giving rise to new, more virulent strains. Alternatively, the virus could combine its genetic material with that from other influenza viruses that already infect humans. The more frequently humans come into contact with infected poultry, the more likely this is to happen.

Both avian and human influenza viruses can also infect certain animals, such as pigs. This creates a genetic 'melting pot' in which viruses can swap their genes and acquire each other's properties. For example, if a bird flu virus were to swap genes with a human flu virus, it could acquire the capacity to infect humans, and this could lead to human-to-human transmission. This could generate a new virus that would pose a greater threat to human health.

The bird flu virus responsible for the recent outbreaks in Asia has been found to be resistant to the two oldest and cheapest flu drugs available, namely rimantidine and amantidine. However, researchers with Australia's Commonwealth Scientific and Industrial Research Organisation (CSIRO) claim that the flu drugs Relenza (zanamivir) and Tamiflu (oseltamivir) are effective treatments against the disease.

There is a worry, however, that antiviral drugs are expensive and in limited supply and that they may not be as effective as hoped if the virus mutates or evolves. In addition, a number of companies are trying to develop a vaccine against bird flu. Such vaccines again present a particular challenge, as the flu viruses against which they are intended to provide protection (by stimulating the production of virus-fighting antibodies) mutate frequently. As a result, any vaccine against a flu virus needs to be modified as the virus itself evolves.

Despite growing concern, experts advise us not to panic about the potential threat of bird flu. Health officials around the world are working together to try to make sure that bird flu doesn't spread and to keep people safe if it does. In an effort to keep bird flu from spreading, authorities in countries that have experienced outbreaks have destroyed millions and millions of birds. The World Health Organization (WHO) is closely monitoring the countries where there have been outbreaks to see if the virus spreads or mutates in a way that makes it more threatening to people. The WHO has created an emergency plan to handle a pandemic, including stockpiling antiviral medications to help people if they do become infected.

In most places, there is no immediate threat to humans from bird flu. The best way to protect yourself is to follow the immune boosting guidelines in this book. If you are in a country where there has been a bird flu outbreak, avoid any contact with chickens, ducks, geese, pigeons, turkeys, quail and any wild birds. Stay away from live bird markets, local poultry farms and any other settings where there might be infected poultry. Avoid touching surfaces that could have been contaminated by the saliva or faeces or urine of birds.

SARS

Severe acute respiratory syndrome, or SARS, is a serious form of pneumonia, resulting in acute respiratory distress and sometimes death. The hallmark symptoms are fever greater than 38°C (100.4°F) and cough, difficulty breathing or other respiratory symptoms. It is a dramatic example of how quickly an infectious disease can spread as a result of world travel. It is also a dramatic example of how quickly governments can act to contain and control disease.

SARS was first identified on 3 February 2003 by WHO physician Dr Carlo Urbani. Within 6 weeks of its discovery, it had infected thousands and killed hundreds of people around the world, including people in Asia, Australia, Europe, Africa, and North and South America. Schools were closed throughout Hong Kong and Singapore. National economies were affected.

The WHO identified SARS as a global health threat and issued an unprecedented travel advisory. Daily WHO updates tracked the spread of SARS 7 days a week. It wasn't clear whether SARS would become a global pandemic, or would settle into a less aggressive pattern.

The rapid, global public health response helped to stem the spread of the virus, and by June 2003, the epidemic had subsided to the degree that on 7 June of that year the WHO backed off from its daily reports. Nevertheless, even as the number of new cases dwindled and travel advisories began to be lifted, the sober truth remained: every new case had the potential to spark another outbreak. Although it can be contained, SARS appears to be here to stay and to have changed the way that the world responds to infectious diseases in the era of widespread international travel.

The flu

The flu is a contagious infection of the nose, throat and lungs caused by the influenza virus. It usually begins abruptly with a fever of between 39°C and 41°C (about 102–106°F). (Adults typically have a lower fever than children.) Other common symptoms include a flushed face, body aches and lack of energy. Some people have dizziness or vomiting. The fever usually lasts for a day or two, but can last 5 days. Somewhere between day 2 and day 4 of the illness, the 'whole body' symptoms begin to subside and respiratory symptoms begin to increase. The flu virus can settle anywhere in the respiratory tract, producing symptoms of a cold, croup, sore throat, ear infection or pneumonia.

The most prominent of the respiratory symptoms is usually a dry, hacking cough. Most people also develop a sore throat and headache. Nasal discharge (runny nose) and sneezing are common. These symptoms (except the cough) usually disappear within 4–7 days. Sometimes, the fever returns. Cough and tiredness usually last for weeks after the rest of the illness is over.

The flu usually arrives in the winter months. The most common way to catch the flu is by breathing in droplets from coughs or sneezes. Less often, it is spread when you touch a surface such as a tap or phone that has the virus on it, and then touch your own mouth, nose or eyes.

Symptoms appear 1–7 days later (usually within 2–3 days). Because the flu virus is airborne and very contagious, with a short incubation period, it often strikes a community all at once. This creates a cluster of school and work absences. Within 2 or 3 weeks of its arrival in a school, much of the classroom might have it.

Millions of people in Europe and the USA get the flu each year. Most recover within a week or two, but some get sick enough to be hospitalized, and several thousand die each year from the flu. Anyone at any age can have serious complications from the flu, but those at highest risk include people over 50 years of age, children aged 6–23 months, women more than 3 months pregnant during the flu season, and anyone with chronic heart, lung or kidney conditions, diabetes or a weakened immune system.

Sometimes people confuse a cold with the flu, since these infections share some of the same symptoms and typically occur at the same time of the year. However, the two diseases are very different. Most people get a cold several times each year but get the flu only once every few years. People often use the term 'stomach flu' to describe a viral in which vomiting or diarrhoea are the main symptoms. This is something of a myth, because the stomach symptoms are not caused by the flu virus. Flu infections are primarily respiratory infections.

Treatment

If you have mild flu and are not at high risk, take these steps: rest, take medicines that relieve symptoms and help you to rest, drink plenty of liquids, avoid aspirin (especially teenagers and children), avoid alcohol and tobacco, and avoid antibiotics (unless necessary for another illness).

If the flu is diagnosed within 48 hours of when symptoms begin, especially if you are at high risk of complications, antiviral medications may help shorten the length of symptoms by approximately 1 day. Medications to treat influenza include amantadine or rimantadine, oseltamivir (Tamiflu) and zanamivir (Relenza). Each of these medicines has different side-effects and affects different viruses. Your doctor will determine which one is best for you. In most people who are otherwise healthy, the flu goes away within 7–10 days.

There are many self-help measures you can take to help to prevent the common cold and flu and other kinds of infections caused by microbial invaders that try to make it past your immune system. You can find all the information and advice you need later in the book, but first let's take a look at what can happen when the immune system doesn't function as it should and things go seriously wrong.

3

Immune system disorders

As well as being more susceptible to colds and flu, a poorly functioning immune system could also increase the risk of allergic disorders and of autoimmune disease, such as type 1 diabetes or rheumatoid arthritis, in which the immune system attacks normal body cells. Other viruses, such as the human immunodeficiency virus (HIV) can also cause the immune system to fail. Even allergies are an example of an immune response gone awry. In general, medical researchers break down disorders of the immune system into four main categories: autoimmune disorders, immunodeficiencies, allergic disorders and cancers of the immune system.

Autoimmune disorders

It is estimated that as many as one in five people suffers from some form of autoimmune disorder. Autoimmune disorders develop when the immune system destroys normal body tissues. This is caused by a hypersensitive reaction, similar to an allergic reaction, where the immune system reacts to a substance that it normally would ignore. In allergies, the immune system reacts to an external substance that would normally be harmless. With autoimmune disorders, however, the immune system reacts to internal or normal 'self' body tissues.

Normally, the immune system is capable of differentiating 'self' from 'non-self' tissue but when the normal control process is disrupted autoimmune disorders occur. They may also occur if normal body tissue is altered so that it is no longer recognized as 'self'. The mechanisms that cause disrupted control or tissue changes are not known. One theory holds that various micro-organisms and drugs may trigger some of these changes, particularly in people with a genetic predisposition to an autoimmune disorder. Many research- ers suspect they occur following infection with an organism that looks similar to particular proteins in the body, which are later mistaken for the organism and wrongly targeted for attack.

Autoimmune disorders typically cause the destruction of one or more types of body tissues, resulting in decreased functioning of an organ or tissue (for example, the islet cells of the pancreas are destroyed in diabetes), abnormal growth of an organ (for example, thyroid enlargement in Grave's disease), or changes in organ function. The disorder may affect only one organ or tissue type or it may affect multiple organs and tissues.

In short, in autoimmune disease, the body's immune defences are turned against the body and rogue immune cells attack tissues. Antibodies may be produced that can react against the body's blood cells, organs and tissues. These antibodies lead immune cells to attack the affected systems, producing a chronic (long-term) disease.

A person may experience more than one autoimmune disorder at the same time. Examples of autoimmune (or autoimmune-related) are discussed below.

Hashimoto's thyroiditis

Hashimoto's thyroiditis is an inflammation of the thyroid gland that most commonly occurs in middle-aged women. It frequently results in hypothyroidism (lowered thyroid function).

Symptoms include intolerance to cold, weight gain, fatigue, constipation, an enlarged neck or the presence of goitre, a small or atrophic thyroid gland (late in the disease), dry skin, hair loss, heavy and irregular menstrual bleeding and difficulty concentrating or thinking.

Pernicious anaemia

Pernicious anaemia is caused by the lack of a substance needed to absorb vitamin B12 from the gastrointestinal tract. This lack of absorption causes anaemia, a condition in which red blood cells are not providing adequate oxygen to body tissues. Other problems related to low levels of vitamin B12 also occur: many cells apart from red blood cells need vitamin B12. These cells include nerve cells, and inadequate levels of vitamin B12 gradually affects sensory and motor nerves, causing neurological problems to develop over time. The anaemia also affects the gastrointestinal system and the cardiovascular system.

The following symptoms may indicate pernicious anaemia: shortness of breath, fatigue, pallor, a rapid heart rate, loss of appetite, diarrhoea, tingling and numbness of hands and feet, sore mouth, unsteady gait (especially in the dark), tongue problems, an impaired sense of smell and bleeding gums.

Addison's disease

Addison's disease is a hormone deficiency caused by damage to the outer layer of the adrenal gland (the adrenal cortex). Symptoms include: extreme weakness; fatigue; unintentional weight loss;

nausea and vomiting; chronic diarrhoea; loss of appetite; darkening of the skin with a patchy skin colour, although paleness may also occur; sores on the inside of a cheek; slow, sluggish, lethargic movement; changes in the blood pressure or heart rate; and a craving for salt.

Type 1 diabetes

Type 1 diabetes is a lifelong disease that occurs when the pancreas produces too little insulin to regulate blood sugar levels appropriately. Symptoms can include: increased thirst, increased urination, weight loss despite increased appetite, nausea, vomiting, abdominal pain, fatigue and absence of menstruation.

Rheumatoid arthritis

Rheumatoid arthritis is a chronic (long-term) disease that causes inflammation of the joints and surrounding tissues. It can also affect other organs. The disease usually begins gradually with fatigue, morning stiffness (lasting more than 1 hour), widespread muscle aches, loss of appetite and weakness. Eventually, joint pain appears. When the joint is not used for a while, it can become warm, tender, and stiff. When the lining of the joint becomes inflamed, it gives off more fluid than usual and the joint becomes swollen. Joint pain is often felt on both sides of the body, and may affect the wrist, knees, elbows, fingers, toes, ankle or neck.

Systemic lupus erythematosus

Systemic lupus erythematosus (SLE) is a chronic, inflammatory autoimmune disorder. It may affect the skin, joints and kidneys as well as other organs. It may occur at any age, but it appears most often in people between the ages of 10 and 50. SLE may also be caused by certain drugs. When this occurs, it is known as drug-induced lupus erythematosus and it is usually reversible when the medication is stopped.

The course of the disease may vary from a mild episodic illness to a severe fatal disease. Symptoms also vary widely in a particular person over time and are characterized by periods of remission and exacerbation. At its onset, only one organ system may be involved. Additional organs may become involved later. Symptoms can include: fever, fatigue, general discomfort, uneasiness or an 'ill feeling' (malaise), weight loss, skin rash (typically a butterfly-shaped rash on the face) that is aggravated by sunlight, joint pain and joint swelling, arthritis, swollen lymph nodes, muscle aches, chest pain, blood in the urine, coughing up blood, nosebleed, swallowing difficulties, numbness and tingling, mouth sores, hair loss, abdominal pain and visual disturbance.

Dermatomyositis

Dermatomyositis is a connective tissue disease that is characterized by inflammation of the muscles and the skin. It can affect people at any age, but most commonly occurs in adults aged 40–60 or in children aged 5–15. It affects women much more often than men. Muscle weakness may appear suddenly or occur slowly over weeks or months. There may be difficulty with raising the arms over the head, rising from a sitting position, and climbing stairs. A dusky, purplish red rash may appear over the face, neck, shoulders, upper chest and back. Joint pain, inflammation of the heart, and lung disease may occur.

Sjögren's syndrome

Sjögren's syndrome is an inflammatory disorder characterized by dry mouth, decreased tear production by the eyes, and other dry mucous membranes. The cause of Sjögren's syndrome, which affects some 3 per cent of the population, is unknown. The syndrome occurs most often in women aged 40–50. It is rare in children, who usually present with another autoimmune disorder before developing the signs of Sjögren's syndrome. Dryness of the eyes and mouth are the most common symptoms of this syndrome; they may occur alone, or with symptoms associated with rheumatoid arthritis or other connective tissue diseases. There may be an associated enlargement of the salivary glands.

Symptoms include: dry or itching eyes, dryness of the mouth, difficulty swallowing, loss of sense of taste, severe dental cavities, hoarseness, fatigue, joint pain or joint swelling, swollen lymph nodes and cloudy corneas.

Multiple sclerosis

Multiple sclerosis (MS) is an autoimmune disease that affects the central nervous system (the brain and spinal cord). MS most commonly begins between the ages of 20 and 40, but it can strike at any age. The exact cause is not known, but MS is believed to result from damage to the myelin sheath – the protective material that surrounds nerve cells. It is a progressive disease, meaning that the damage gets worse over time. Inflammation destroys the myelin, leaving multiple areas of scar tissue (sclerosis). The inflammation

21

occurs when the body's own immune cells attack the nervous system. The inflammation causes nerve impulses to slow down or become blocked, leading to the symptoms of MS which include: weakness of one or more extremities, paralysis of one or more extremities, tremor of one or more extremities, muscle spasticity (uncontrollable spasm of muscle groups), numbness or abnormal sensation in any area, tingling and facial pain. Repeated episodes, or flare-ups, of inflammation can also occur in any area of the brain and spinal cord.

Myasthenia gravis

Myasthenia gravis is a neuromuscular disorder characterized by variable weakness of voluntary muscles, which often improves with rest and worsens with activity. The condition is caused by an abnormal immune response.

Reiter's syndrome

Reiter's syndrome is a group of symptoms consisting of arthritis (inflammation of the joints), urethritis (inflammation of the urethra), conjunctivitis (inflammation of the lining of the eye), and sores on the skin and mucous membranes. The risk factors for the syndrome include infection with certain bacteria (*Chlamydia, Campylobacter, Salmonella* or *Yersinia*), being male and aged under 40, and (possibly) a genetic predisposition. The disorder is rare in younger children, but it may occur in adolescents.

Grave's disease

Grave's disease is an autoimmune disease that causes overactivity of the thyroid gland (hyperthyroidism). The production of thyroid hormone is increased, causing a wide range of symptoms from anxiety and restlessness to insomnia and weight loss. In addition, the eyeballs may begin to protrude causing irritation and increased tear production. Grave's disease is caused by inappropriate immune system activation that targets the thyroid gland and causes overproduction of thyroid hormones. Risk factors include being a woman aged over 20, although the disorder may occur at any age and may affect men.

Chronic fatigue syndrome

Chronic fatigue syndrome (CFS) is a condition of prolonged and severe tiredness or weariness (fatigue) that is not relieved by rest and is not directly caused by other conditions. To be diagnosed with chronic fatigue syndrome, the tiredness must be severe enough to decrease ability to participate in ordinary activities by 50 per cent. The exact cause of CFS is unknown. Some researchers suspect it may be caused by a virus, such as Epstein–Barr virus or human herpes virus-6 (HHV-6). However, no distinct viral cause has been identified. Recent studies have shown that CFS may be caused by inflammation of pathways in the nervous system, and that this inflammation may be some sort of immune response or autoimmune process. CFS may occur when a viral illness is complicated by an inadequate or dysfunctional immune response. Other factors such as age, prior illness, stress, environment or genetic disposition may also play a role. CFS most commonly occurs in adults aged between 30 and 50. Symptoms of CFS are similar to those of most common viral infections (muscle aches, headache and fatigue); the symptoms often develop within a few hours or days and last for 6 months or more.

Treatment of autoimmune disorders

Autoimmunity is typically controlled through balanced suppression of the immune system. The goal of medical treatment is to reduce the immune response against normal body tissue while leaving intact the immune response against micro-organisms and abnormal tissues. Corticosteroids and immunosuppressant medications (including cyclophosphamide and azathioprine) are used to reduce the immune response.

The symptoms are treated according to the type and severity. Hormones or other substances normally produced by the affected organ may need to be supplemented. This may, for example, include thyroid supplements, vitamins, insulin injections or other supplements. Disorders that affect the blood components may require blood transfusions. Measures to assist mobility or other functions may be needed for disorders that affect the bones, joints or muscles.

The outcome of treatment varies with the specific disorder. Most autoimmune disorders are chronic, but many can be controlled with treatment. Side-effects of medications used to suppress the immune system can be severe. Some patients find that natural or alternative medicines used alongside treatment from their doctor can offer relief.

Immunodeficiency disorders

Immunodeficiencies occur when a part of the immune system is not present or is not working properly. Sometimes a person is born with an immunodeficiency – these immunodeficiencies are called primary immunodeficiencies – although symptoms of the disorder may not show up until later in life. Immunodeficiencies can also be acquired through infection or produced by drugs. These are called secondary or acquired immunodeficiencies.

Immunodeficiency can cause persistent or recurrent infections, severe infections by organisms that are normally mild, incomplete recovery from illness or a poor response to treatment, and an increased incidence of cancer and other tumours. Immunodeficiency disorders may affect any part of the immune system. Most commonly, they cause decreased functioning of T or B lymphocytes (or both) or deficient antibody production.

Malnutrition, particularly with lack of protein, may cause immunodeficiency. Acquired immunodeficiency may also be a complication of diseases such as HIV infection and AIDS.

HIV–AIDS is a disease that slowly and steadily destroys the immune system. It is caused by HIV, a virus that wipes out certain types of lymphocytes called T-helper cells. Without T-helper cells, the immune system is unable to defend the body against normally harmless organisms, which can cause life-threatening infections in people who have AIDS. Babies can get HIV infection from their mother while in the uterus, during the birth process or during breastfeeding. People can get HIV infection by having unprotected sexual intercourse with an infected person or from sharing contaminated needles for drugs, steroids or tattoos.

Immunodeficiencies can also be caused by medications. There are several medicines that suppress the immune system. One of the drawbacks of chemotherapy treatment for cancer, for example, is that it attacks not only cancer cells but also other fast-growing, healthy cells, including those found in the bone marrow and other parts of the immune system. In addition, people with autoimmune disorders or people who have had organ transplants may need to take immunosuppressant medications. These medicines can also reduce the ability of the immune system to fight infections and can cause secondary immunodeficiency.

Persistent or recurrent infections, or severe infections caused by micro-organisms that do not usually cause severe infection, may be clues that an immunodeficiency disorder is present. Other clues include a poor response to treatment; delayed or incomplete recovery from illness; the presence of certain types of cancers, such as Kaposi's sarcoma or non-Hodgkins lymphoma; and certain opportunistic infections, such as *Pneumocystis carinii* pneumonia (PCP; also known as *Pneumocystis jeroveci* pneumonia) or recurrent fungal yeast infections.

Treatment of immunodeficiency disorders

The goal of treatment for immunodeficiency disorders includes protection against (and treatment of) diseases and infections. Any illness or infection is treated aggressively in patients with immunosuppression. This may involve prolonged use of antimicrobial medications (such as antibiotics or antifungal medications), the use of powerful antimicrobial medications to treat any infection, and preventive (prophylactic) treatments.

Interferon, which is used to treat viral infections and some types of cancer, and zidovudine (also known as AZT), which is used to treat AIDS, are two immunostimulant drugs (medications that increase the efficiency of the immune system). Persons with HIV and AIDS may take combinations of drugs to reduce the amount of virus in their immune systems, thus improving their immunity.

Bone marrow transplant may be used to treat certain immunodeficiency conditions. Passive immunity (administration of antibodies produced by another person or animal) may occasionally be recommended to prevent illness after exposure to a micro-organism.

Some immunodeficiency disorders are mild and result in occasional illness. Others are severe and may be fatal. Immunosuppression that results from medications is often reversible once the medication is stopped. There is no known prevention for congenital immunodeficiency disorders. Safe sex practices and avoiding the sharing of body fluids may help to prevent HIV infection and AIDS. Good nutrition may prevent acquired immunodeficiency caused by malnutrition.

Allergic disorders

Allergic disorders occur when the immune system over-reacts to exposure to antigens (such as invading micro-organisms) in the environment. The substances that provoke such attacks are called allergens. The immune response can cause symptoms such as swelling, watery eyes and sneezing, and even a life-threatening reaction called anaphylaxis. Taking medications called antihistamines can relieve most symptoms.

Some examples of allergic disorders are discussed below.

Asthma

Asthma is a respiratory disorder that can cause breathing problems and frequently involves an allergic response by the lungs. If the lungs are oversensitive to certain allergens (such as pollen, moulds, animal dander or dust mites), the reaction can trigger the breathing tubes in the lungs to become narrowed, leading to reduced airflow and making it hard for a person to breathe. Asthma symptoms can also be triggered by respiratory infections, exercise, cold air, tobacco smoke and other pollutants, stress, foods, or drug allergies. Aspirin and other non-steroidal anti-inflammatory medications (NSAIDS) provoke asthma in some patients.

Most people with asthma have periodic wheezing attacks separated by symptom-free periods. Asthma occurs in 3–5 per cent of adults and 7–10 per cent of children. Half of the people with asthma develop it before the age of 10, and almost all develop it before the age of 30. Asthma symptoms can decrease over time, especially in children. Medical treatment is aimed at avoiding known allergens and respiratory irritants and at controlling symptoms and airway inflammation through medication, taken by mouth through an inhaler. Allergens can sometimes be identified by noting which substances cause an allergic reaction.

Eczema

Eczema, also known as atopic dermatitis, causes a scaly, itchy rash. A hypersensitivity reaction occurs in the skin, causing chronic inflammation. The inflammation causes the skin to become itchy and scaly. Chronic irritation and scratching can cause the skin to thicken and become leathery in texture. Although atopic dermatitis is not necessarily caused by an allergic reaction, it more often occurs in people who have allergies, hay fever or asthma or in those who have a family history of these conditions. Eczema is most common in infants, and at least half of those cases clear by the age of 3 years. In adults, it is generally a chronic or recurring condition.

Exposure to environmental irritants can worsen symptoms, as can dryness of the skin, exposure to water, temperature changes, and stress. Consult your doctor for a diagnosis of eczema because it can be difficult to differentiate from other skin disorders. Treatment should be guided by your doctor.

Allergies

Environmental allergies (to dust mites, for example), seasonal allergies (such as hay fever), drug allergies (reactions to specific medications or drugs), food allergies (such as to nuts) and allergies to toxins (bee stings, for example) are other common conditions people usually refer to as allergies. The allergy is caused by an oversensitive immune system, which leads to a misdirected immune response when the immune system reacts to substances (allergens) that are generally harmless and in most people do not cause an immune response.

When an allergen enters the body of a person with a sensitized immune system, histamine and other chemicals are released by certain cells. This causes itching, swelling, mucus production, muscle spasms, hives, skin rashes and other symptoms.

Symptoms vary in severity from person to person. Most people have symptoms that cause discomfort without being life-threatening. A few people have life-threatening reactions (called anaphylaxis). Of course, the best 'treatment' is to avoid whatever causes your allergies in the first place. It may be impossible to avoid everything you are allergic to completely, but you can often take steps to reduce your exposure. This is especially important for food and drug allergies. Medications, such as antihistamines, can also be used to treat allergies.

Cancers of the immune system

Cancer occurs when cells grow out of control. This can also happen with the cells of the immune system. For example, lymphoma involves the lymphoid tissues and is one of the more common childhood cancers. Leukaemia, which involves abnormal overgrowth of leucocytes, is another common cancer of the immune system. These rare disorders can be treated – some of them very successfully – by drugs or irradiation.

Summary

As noted above, a large number of health problems are related to immune system dysfunction. On the surface, these conditions seem to be quite different. For instance, the symptoms of rheumatoid arthritis (inflamed, painful joints and limited mobility) are different from those of Crohn's disease (chronic diarrhoea, abdominal pain and fever) and different again from those of asthma (coughing, wheezing.) Yet, as different as these conditions seem to be from each other, they are all caused or triggered by an immune system that for some reason isn't functioning properly and is struggling to cope with the pressures placed upon it.

The next chapter takes a look at some common reasons why the immune system may be struggling or not functioning as efficiently as it could be, and also at early warning signs of an immune system in trouble.

4

Heeding your body's warning signals

Even though your immune system is invisible, there are ways to find out if it is in trouble if you know what to look out for.

You can start by thinking about how you feel right now? If you feel good that's amazing, as at this very second there are millions of microscopic invaders just waiting for an opportunity to attack and make you ill, and the only thing that stands in their way is your immune system. If you don't feel so good, if you have the odd ache or pain or just feel tired, fed up and run down, don't ignore those feelings. Take the time to listen to what your body is trying to tell you.

Your body will tell you if your immune system is in danger. It is important to listen to it and be aware of any slight changes because the earlier you recognize the signs and symptoms of weakened immunity the faster you can take corrective action and the more likely you are to avoid becoming ill. Use the checklist below to see if you need to give your immune system a boost.

Is your immune system in trouble?

Answer yes or no to the questions below:

- Hair: Does it lack shine? Is it dull or greasy or thinning?
- Head: Do you suffer from recurring headaches or bouts of fogginess and dizziness? Does your head feel heavy and sore?
- Eyes: Do your eyes feel tired? Are they bloodshot or itchy? Are they dull, not sparkling?
- Ears: Can you sometimes hear a high-pitched noise? Are your ears itchy or painful?
- Nose: Is your nose runny, congested or itchy? Do you sneeze? Is there a loss of smell?
- Mouth: Does your breath smell bad? Do you have a bad taste in your mouth? Is your tongue sore or swollen? Do you suffer from bleeding gums and or mouth ulcers? Do you have bad teeth or gum disease? Is there loss of taste? Are your lips cracked and sore? Do you often get cold sores?
- Neck: Is your neck stiff and sore when you move?
- Throat: Is your throat itchy or sore? Do you sometimes have difficulty swallowing?

- Digestive tract: Do you suffer from indigestion, gas, diarrhoea, bloating, constipation or abdominal pain? Do you feel nauseated at certain times of the day?
- Muscles: Do your muscles feel weak and tingly? Do you get injuries easily?
- Joints: Are your joints stiff and painful?
- Skin: Do you have spots or rashes? Is your skin dry, dull or bloated? Do you have body odour problems?
- Nails: Do you have white spots, ridges, splits or blue tinges on your nails?
- Energy levels: Do you need coffee or other stimulants, like chocolate or sugar, to keep going? Are your energy levels intermittent, erratic or non existent? Do you feel tired a lot of the time? Do you yawn a lot during the day? Do you often feel apathetic?
- Sleep: Are you having trouble sleeping? Do you sweat excessively in the night?
- Brain power: Do you find it hard to concentrate? Are you forgetful? Is your memory poor?
- Feelings: Do you feel stressed, depressed, sad, up-and-down, irritable or just below par?
- Hunger: Do you get food cravings or feelings of intense hunger? Or are you off your food?
- Lifestyle: Are you overweight? Do you smoke? Is your job sedentary? Do you take very little exercise? Do you spend little time in natural daylight? Do you eat a lot of refined, processed or convenience foods? Is your diet high in sugar?
- General health: Do you get more than three colds a year? Do you find it hard to get over an infection? Do you suffer from repeated infections? Do you have allergies? Are you prone to thrush or cystitis? Do you suffer from anaemia? Do wounds heal slowly? Do you feel the cold more than other people? Are your periods irregular? Have you noticed a loss of libido? Do you feel as if you've lost your 'va-va-voom'?

If you find that you are answering 'yes' more than 'no' to the questions above and you can't find a logical explanation (for example, a stiff neck is normal if you've slept in an awkward position, ravenous hunger is normal after a long walk in the countryside), the chances are your immune system needs some help. This book can give you guidance in the chapters that follow.

If you answered mainly 'no' to the questions above, your immune system is doing its job well. To fine-tune your health, take note of any 'yes' answers and find ways to turn them into 'no' answers. Again this book can show you how.

Immunity enemies at a glance

The first step to making sure your immune system stays reasonably strong is to know your enemies (i.e. the factors that can hamper your immune system). Although a number of disorders, some genetic, are linked to improper immune function, the most common causes of weakened immunity are, in fact, related to diet and lifestyle.

Listed below are common lifestyle factors that research has shown can depress your immune system and put your health at risk:

- Poor diet
- Lack of essential nutrients in the diet
- Stress
- Depression
- Lack of sleep
- Smoking
- Lack of exercise
- Excessive intake of alcohol
- Pesticides, chemicals and food additives
- Overuse of antibiotics
- Poor living habits

Each immunity enemy listed above is explored in more detail later, but at this stage it is important to point out that the immune system can be weakened by factors within your control as well as accidents, medication and immunodeficiency diseases. In fact, in the great majority of cases you are directly responsible for the weakness of your immune system.

Even the most susceptible person can boost the immune system by heeding the warning signs of a weakened immune system, taking better care of himself or herself and getting immunized if eligible. These measures will not completely prevent you from getting sick, but they will help. And when you do catch that unavoidable yearly bug, its effects will not be as strong or drawn out as you might expect.

The remaining chapters of this book explain the many ways in which you can take control of your health and boost your immunity.

First, what your doctor can offer you and the pros and cons of vaccinations and treatments for immune disorders is discussed. Then, a simple, practical, but incredibly potent, self-help action plan designed to boost your immunity is outlined – not only will the action plan help to keep you free from disease but it will also help you to feel great, to perform better, to look good and to live longer

5

What your doctor can offer you

Your doctor can help you to stay healthy by offering you appropriate vaccinations to prevent disease and medications to treat them.

Vaccination

Vaccination is believed to be your best line of defence against certain diseases. Many vaccines are given in childhood, but adults can also be routinely vaccinated to prevent some illnesses, such as tetanus and influenza. Currently, vaccines for nearly two dozen different diseases are licensed for use in Europe and the USA. Twelve of these vaccines are recommended for children under the age of 2 years. According to the US Centers for Disease Control and Prevention, widespread and persistent immunization efforts have lowered the incidence rates of several serious illnesses, including diphtheria, tetanus, measles and polio, by more than 95 per cent since the beginning of the 20th century.

Vaccines work by stimulating your body's immune system. Your body can become immune to bacteria, viruses and other germs by actually getting a disease (natural immunity) but it can also become immune through vaccines (vaccine-induced immunity). Natural immunity results after you've been exposed naturally to a specific virus or bacterium, so that the next time you encounter it, antibodies and memory T cells go to work. They immediately react to the organism, attacking it before disease can develop. Your immune system can recognize and effectively combat thousands of different organisms.

The immunity that you develop following vaccination is similar to the immunity that is acquired from natural infection. The vaccine contains a killed or weakened form or a derivative of the infectious germ, and this triggers your immune system's infection-fighting ability and memory without exposure to the actual disease-producing germs. The vaccine makes your body think that it's being invaded by a specific organism and so your immune system goes to work to destroy the invader and prevent it from infecting you again. If you're exposed to a disease for which you've been vaccinated, the invading germs are met by antibodies that will destroy them.

Several doses of a vaccine may be needed for a full immune response. In addition, the immunity provided by some vaccines, such as the tetanus vaccine, isn't lifelong – because the immune response may decrease over time, you may need another dose of a vaccine (a booster shot) to restore or increase your immunity.

Note that vaccines, like prescription drugs, aren't completely free of possible side-effects. Most effects are minor and temporary, such as a sore arm, mild fever or swelling at the injection site. Serious side-effects, such as a seizure or a high fever, are extremely rare.

Types of vaccines

Vaccines are prepared in several different ways. For each type, the goal is the same – to stimulate an immune response without causing disease.

Live, weakened vaccines

Some vaccines, such as those for measles, mumps and chickenpox (varicella), use live viruses that have been weakened (or attenuated). This type of vaccine results in a strong antibody response, sometimes making only one dose necessary to establish lifelong immunity.

Inactivated vaccines

Other vaccines use killed (inactivated) bacteria or viruses. The inactivated polio vaccine is made this way. These vaccines are generally safer than live vaccines because the disease organisms can't mutate back into a disease-causing state once they've been killed.

Toxoid vaccines

Some types of bacteria cause disease by producing toxins that invade the bloodstream. Toxoid vaccines, such as those for diphtheria and tetanus, use bacterial toxin that has been rendered harmless to provide immunity to the toxin.

Acellular and subunit vaccines

Acellular and subunit vaccines are made by using only part of the virus or bacteria. The vaccines against hepatitis and *Haemophilus influenzae* type b are made in this way.

Vaccine-induced immunity versus natural immunity: which is better?

Gaining natural immunity involves considerable risk. Diseases that are preventable by vaccination can kill or cause permanent disability – for example, paralysis from polio, deafness from meningitis, liver damage from hepatitis B, or brain damage (encephalitis) from measles. Immunity from a vaccine offers protection similar to that acquired by natural infection. At the same time, vaccines rarely put people at risk of the serious complications of infection.

Some people argue that immunity from vaccines isn't effective. It's true that vaccines aren't 100 per cent protective. Most childhood vaccines are effective for 85–95 per cent of recipients. However, should there be a disease outbreak, those who have been immunized usually have a less serious illness, while those who have not been are in the greatest danger.

Immunization is one of the best ways you can protect yourself and your children against infectious disease. By stimulating your body's natural resistance to disease, thereby creating immunity, vaccines are your first line of defence against the likes of polio, measles, mumps, rubella, influenza, tetanus and diphtheria. Were it not for the widespread use of vaccines a far greater number of deaths would occur during childhood and many more people would be living with chronic and often crippling after-effects of disease.

In 1979, the WHO announced the success of a 10-year programme to eradicate smallpox. Smallpox had been a devastating disease for centuries. It killed 30 per cent of those who were infected. Most survivors were left with disfiguring scars. Many were blinded from corneal scarring. The success of the smallpox campaign increased efforts to immunize against other infectious diseases. Most notable is the Global Polio Eradication Initiative. At the time the programme was launched in 1988, polio was widespread, with cases reported in 125 countries. Only six countries reported widespread polio as of June 2005. Efforts remain under way to achieve a polio-free world by the end of the decade. Within Europe and the USA, vaccines have reduced the incidence of measles and diphtheria by 98 per cent.

If you weigh up the pros and cons, immunization, for yourself and your children, is probably the right thing to do because it protects you as well as others. Infectious diseases that have virtually disappeared in Europe and the USA can quickly reappear if international travellers unintentionally carry the disease. From a single entry point, an infectious disease can spread quickly, particularly among those who are unprotected.

Vaccine safety concerns

Despite the success of vaccines and the advice from doctors, there is public concern about the safety of vaccination. Hearing or seeing media reports regarding a sickness or severe reaction of a child who has just been immunized can raise levels of concern.

Many adults fear that introducing a vaccine into themselves or their children may trigger serious side-effects or even cause the disease itself. The debate as to the safety of the measles–mumps–rubella (MMR) vaccination highlighted this fear, even though there is a large body of evidence and research to suggest that MMR vaccination is safe.

It is important to point out that before vaccines can be used, they must meet strict safety standards established by bodies such as the US Food and Drug Administration (FDA). Meeting these standards requires a lengthy development process that can take up to 10 years. Vaccines are also subject to ongoing research and review by doctors, researchers and public health officials. Compared with other pharmaceutical products, vaccines require higher standards of safety because they are usually given to healthy people to prevent disease in the individual and in society in general.

If you have any concerns about vaccinations that you or your child are eligible for, it is important that you discuss them with your doctor so that you can come to an informed decision. You can also look at the following website: http://www.immunisation.nhs.uk, a comprehensive, up-to-date and accurate source of information on vaccines, disease and immunization in the UK.

Flu jab

Flu is a highly infectious illness that spreads very rapidly by coughs and sneezes from people who are already carrying the virus. Catching flu is a nasty experience for most people. But for some people it can lead to really serious illnesses like bronchitis and pneumonia, which may mean they need hospital treatment. Many, mainly older, people die from influenza every winter.

See your doctor about the flu jab if you're aged 65 years or over or if you have any of the following problems (however

---

old you are): a serious heart or chest complaint, including serious asthma; serious kidney or liver disease; diabetes; lowered immunity caused by disease or treatment such as corticosteroid medication or cancer treatment. Your doctor may also advise you to have the flu jab if you are the parent of a child (over the age of 6 months) with a long-term condition – your child's condition may get worse if he or she does catch flu.

If you're the carer of an elderly or disabled person make sure he or she has had a flu jab. You should also get the jab yourself if the welfare of the person you care for would be at risk if you fell ill (i.e. you wouldn't be able to look after him or her). Ask your doctor for advice.

The best time to have the flu jab is between late September and early November, ready for the winter. Don't wait until there's a flu epidemic. The flu virus changes, so you need to have a flu jab every year to make sure that you are protected against the latest strain of the virus, which generally appears every winter.

If you think you need a flu vaccination, check with your doctor or the practice nurse. If a nurse visits you regularly, you can ask him or her. Alternatively ask your local pharmacist. Most doctors organize special vaccination sessions in the autumn.

Your body starts making antibodies to the vaccine virus about 7–10 days after the injection, and these antibodies help protect you against any similar viruses you then come into contact with. Flu vaccinations protect against most flu viruses, but they won't stop you catching the many other viruses that appear every winter, and they don't protect against bird flu. Because flu is generally serious, it makes sense to get protected. There is no active virus in a flu vaccine so it can't cause flu. People sometimes catch other flu-like viruses, or very occasionally catch flu before the vaccine takes effect.

Medications

Some medicines can help you from becoming susceptible to infectious agents. For example, taking an anti-parasitic medication might protect you from contracting malaria if you travel to or live in an area where your risk is high. Antihistamines can prevent or reduce allergy symptoms. After exposure to certain organisms, such as those that cause bacterial meningitis, your doctor may prescribe antibiotics to lower your risk of infection or reduce the severity of symptoms. Or you may choose an over-the-counter antibiotic cream or ointment for minor cuts and scrapes. However, long-term, indiscriminate use of antibiotics isn't recommended in most cases. It won't prevent bacterial infections and instead may result in a more resistant, harder-to-treat strain of bacteria when infections do occur.

Antihistamines

Antihistamines, such as chlorpheniramine (Piriton) and loratadine (Clarityn), are most commonly found in medicines for allergic conditions like hay fever. They are also in some cough and cold remedies, some preparations for nausea and some migraine treatments. A number of antihistamine-containing products are available without prescription from a pharmacy ('over-the-counter'). These are generally for use on a temporary basis. Other preparations can only be prescribed by a doctor.

Antihistamines work by blocking the action of histamine at special sites (receptors) in the skin, nose, blood vessels and airways. Histamine is a natural chemical produced by the body in response to foreign organisms and other foreign particles. It is an important part of your immune system but sometimes the body releases too much histamine and this produces the allergic reaction. For example, in hay fever, too much histamine is released in response to pollen and the histamine receptors in the nose are over-stimulated. Histamine causes more blood to flow to the location of contact, and the skin and mucous membranes swell, an itchy feeling arises and fluids are released. All of these things are attempts to get rid of the intruders, which are actually harmless. The nose and the eyes are irritated, causing sneezing, an itchy and runny nose, and red and itchy eyes.

There are two types of antihistamines, the older ones such as chlorpheniramine, which are sedating and have drowsiness as one of their main side-effects and should therefore be avoided in most cases, and the newer, non-sedating ones such as loratadine, which rarely cause drowsiness. Other less common side-effects, from the sedating antihistamines in particular, are headache, difficulty in passing urine, dry mouth, blurred vision, and digestive tract problems such as feeling or being sick, constipation or diarrhoea. Rarely, some antihistamines can also cause palpitations and abnormal heart rhythms, high blood pressure, allergic reactions (with swelling, rash, and breathing difficulties), dizziness and confusion.

Antihistamine preparations applied locally (to the nose, eyes or skin) can cause irritation.

Antihistamines are typically used to relieve the symptoms of allergies like hay fever (seasonal rhinitis) and perennial rhinitis (hay fever-like symptoms all year round); certain allergic rashes such as urticaria (nettle rash); itchy skin (pruritus); and insect bites and stings. Some are also used to treat sickness, particularly motion sickness, as well as dizziness, poor sleep and tickly coughs. This is because some antihistamines have an effect on the part of the brain involved in these reactions and sensations. In the majority of cases, antihistamines, in particular the ones that do not cause drowsiness, are effective and safe to use. In hay fever, the big advantage of antihistamines is that they treat the nose, the eyes and the terrible itching that some sufferers get in the throat or ears. The drawback is that they are not so effective for the blockage in the nose that troubles some people.

The most obvious way to control an allergy is to find out what you are allergic to and then avoid it. This can be possible if it is something obvious that you've touched (like nickel in jewellery) or eaten (like shellfish), but in some cases, such as in hay fever, it can be extremely difficult to avoid pollen – then, antihistamines may be the best alternative. If you have hay fever and don't want to take antihistamines, then stay indoors with the windows shut as much as possible when there is a high pollen count, and avoid newly mown lawns or fields. When you have to go outside, sunglasses can help stop pollen getting in your eyes, and washing your face and hands when you come in can also help.

Immunotherapy

Immunotherapy (commonly called allergy shots) is a treatment to reduce your allergic reaction to allergens (substances to which you are allergic). Research has shown that allergy shots can reduce symptoms of allergic rhinitis (hay fever) and allergic asthma. Allergy shots can be effective against grass, weed and tree pollens, dust mites, cat and dog dander and insect stings. Allergy shots are less effective against moulds and are not a useful method for the treatment of food allergy.

Immunotherapy consists of a series of injections (shots) with a solution that contains the allergens that cause your symptoms. Treatment usually begins with a weak solution given once or twice a week. The strength of the solution is gradually increased with each dose. Once the strongest dosage is reached, the injections are often given once a month to control your symptoms. At this point, you have decreased your sensitivity to the allergens. You have reached your maintenance level. Allergy shots should always be given at your doctor's surgery.

Six months to a year of allergy shots may be required before you notice any improvement in symptoms. If your symptoms do not improve after this time, ask your doctor to review your overall treatment programme. If the treatment is effective, the shots often continue for 3–5 years, until the person is symptom-free or until symptoms can be controlled with mild medications for 1 year. In general, allergy shots should be stopped if they are not effective within 2–3 years.

Are allergy shots safe?

Allergy shots are really like vaccinations: They boost the defences of the immune system to help the body to block the allergic reaction. In the hands of a well-trained and experienced doctor, allergy shots are safe and effective and can be given to children as young as 4 or 5 years old. Allergy shots, which are given year-round, work better against some substances than others. Generally, the shots are most effective against insect venoms and allergens that are inhaled, such as pollens, dust, moulds and animal dander.

Although a shot may seem like an unusual way to treat allergies (why would you want to deliberately inject into your arm the very thing that is making you unwell?) allergy shots are an effective method of decreasing sensitivity to the things that are triggering an allergic reaction.

Allergen immunotherapy isn't necessary for everyone with allergies. Many people get along fine by living in homes that are as free as possible of allergens or by taking allergy medication during their peak allergy season. However, some people suffer from allergies year-round, and some just can't tolerate or are uncomfortable with their medications. Many of these people can greatly benefit from allergen immunotherapy.

There are no long-term complications associated with this form of therapy, but there is a small risk of allergic reactions immediately following the injection. These allergic reactions can be severe and for that reason doctors advise you to remain in their surgery for 20–30 minutes after receiving the shot.

Typically, allergy shots may cause slight swelling or redness at the injection site. These reactions can occur immediately after the injection, or they can occur several hours later. This mild allergic reaction is usually harmless and goes away within 24 hours. The shots may also cause symptoms that are similar to the allergy symptoms you experience: an itchy or stuffy nose, itchy or watery eyes, and sneezing.

Immunosuppressants

Immunosuppressants are powerful medicines that dampen down the activity of the body's immune system. Immunosuppressants are used to prevent rejection of a transplanted organ and to treat autoimmune diseases such as psoriasis, rheumatoid arthritis and Crohn's disease. Some treatments for cancer act as immunosuppressants. Immuno-suppressants can also be helpful for controlling severe eczema because they suppress the overactivity of the immune system that is causing the inflammation in the skin. They are used to treat only very severe eczema that has not responded to treatment with more conventional treatments, such as topical corticosteroids. They are prescribed only by medical specialists.

Antibiotics: a blessing or a curse?

Antibiotics are both a blessing and a curse. They are strong medicines that can stop some life-threatening infections and save lives. But if they aren't used in the right way, antibiotics can do more harm than good.

Antibiotics are drugs used to kill or harm specific bacteria. Since their discovery in the 1930s, antibiotics have made it possible to cure bacterial diseases such as pneumonia, tuberculosis and meningitis, saving the lives of millions of people around the world.

However, antibiotics must be used in the correct way. Because bacteria are living organisms, they are always changing in an effort to resist the drugs that can kill them. Taking antibiotics for colds and other viral illnesses not only won't work, but it also has a dangerous side-effect: over time, this practice has helped to create bacteria that have become more of a challenge to kill. Frequent and inappropriate use of antibiotics selects for strains of bacteria that can resist treatment. This is called bacterial resistance. These resistant bacteria require higher doses of medicine or stronger antibiotics to treat them. Doctors have even found bacteria that are resistant to some of the most powerful antibiotics available today.

Antibiotic resistance is a widespread problem, which the US Centers for Disease Control and Prevention calls 'one of the world's most pressing public health problems'. Bacteria that were once highly responsive to antibiotics have become increasingly resistant.

Among infections that are becoming harder to treat are pneumococcal infections (which cause pneumonia, ear infections, sinus infections and meningitis), skin infections and tuberculosis.

The correct use of these drugs is the best way to ensure that antibiotics remain useful in treating infections. At your doctor's surgery you may well find leaflets explaining that antibiotics are not a miracle cure and detailing the problems and concerns associated with antibiotic use. These concerns include:

• Patients who fail to take the full course of antibiotics prescribed for them. This can aid the rise of drug-resistant germs and is particularly worrying in the case of serious illnesses. In recent years, drug-resistant forms of diseases like tuberculosis have been noted in many countries around the world. These are thought to be a result of patients failing to finish courses of antibiotics. The full course of drugs should be finished so there are no leftovers. A person may feel well, but there may still be bacteria left in the body which could cause a recurrence of the illness.

• Patients who forget to take their antibiotics at the times prescribed. Doctors should explain clearly when and how often the drugs should be taken. They say patients should take their pills at the same time each day to aid memory.

• Some patients think they can share other people's antibiotics or use an unfinished course of antibiotics for another illness. Antibiotics are prescribed for a specific illness and a specific person and should not be shared.

• Patients who suffer from side-effects when taking antibiotics should inform their GP as the dosage may be too high or they may respond better to a different course of antibiotics. Like all drugs, antibiotics have side-effects. One of the most common is antibiotic-associated stomach upsets and diarrhoea (AAD), a potentially serious condition that affects up to 20 per cent of people receiving antibiotic therapy. AAD occurs when antibiotics disturb the natural balance of good and bad bacteria in your intestinal tract, causing harmful bacteria to proliferate far beyond their normal numbers. The result is often frequent, watery bowel movements.

Alternatives to vaccination and medications

Vaccination is a good insurance policy against disease and medications can also be lifesavers. Do bear in mind, though, that neither vaccinations nor medications are miracle cures and the best way to

How do I know when I need antibiotics?

The answer to this question depends on what is causing your infection. The following are some basic guidelines:

- Colds and flu: antibiotics can be effective against infections caused by bacteria, but it is important to point out that they do not work against infections caused by viruses; viruses cause colds and most coughs and sore throats. Don't take antibiotics for colds or the flu. Often, the best thing you can do is to let a cold or the flu run its course. Sometimes this can take 2 weeks or more. Call your doctor if your illness gets worse after 2 weeks.
- Cough or bronchitis: viruses almost always cause these illnesses. However, if you have a problem with your lungs or an illness that lasts a long time, bacteria may actually be the cause. Your doctor may decide to try using an antibiotic.
- Sore throat: most sore throats are caused by viruses and don't need antibiotics. However, strep throat is caused by bacteria. A throat swab for laboratory testing is usually needed before your doctor will prescribe an antibiotic for strep throat.
- Ear infections: there are several types of ear infections, and antibiotics are used for some, but not all, of these.
- Sinus infections: antibiotics can be used to treat some sinus infections. A runny nose and yellow or green mucus do not necessarily mean you need an antibiotic.

safeguard your health against disease is to make sure you and your children have a fighting-fit immune system. Although major factors determining the strength of your immunity include such things as inherited genetics, tendencies to allergies and whether you were breast fed, it's encouraging to know that good nutrition and a positive lifestyle can affect the way your genetic make-up is expressed.

There are many things you can do to help boost your immune system and you'll find them outlined in the self-defence action plan that follows. Not only will these things increase your resistance to illness and allergies, they can also improve your general health and well-being so that you can reap the rewards of a healthy, vigorous life.

6

Building a strong immune system:
your self-defence action plan

As touched on briefly in Chapter 2, your immune system, the complex network of tissues, organs, cells and chemicals that protects your body from infection and illness, has three lines of defence: innate, adaptive and lymphatic. Innate immunity provides an immediate response to the threat of infection, adaptive immunity provides a follow-up response several days later, and your lymphatic system produces and transports the immune cells needed to fight pathogens. When you are aiming to stimulate your immune system into optimal performance you need to consider them all.

The self-defence action plan outlined below involves a series of steps designed to boost all three lines of defence so that you can rebuild your immunity and tip the balance toward health.

Your self-defence action plan involves:

- Eating to boost immunity
- Exercise and skin-brushing techniques
- Balancing hygiene
- Positive thinking and the fighting spirit
- Natural ways to boost your body's defence mechanisms

The diet and lifestyle changes recommended in the plan should not be attempted all at once. To increase your chances of success, tackle one change at a time and take your time. It's very difficult to change everything at once so don't set yourself up to fail. Start slowly and gradually. It typically takes about 3–4 months before you'll see major improvements in your health and well-being, though even after a week or two most people will notice an improvement in their energy levels.

Boosting your immunity isn't about a short-term fix. It's about making changes that will last you for the rest of your life. Small and gradual changes are the best way to create long-term improvements in your health and well-being. The steps are designed to build a strong immune system rather than simply to treat the signs and symptoms of poor immunity.

Fatigue, lethargy, repeated infections, slow wound healing,

allergies, thrush, colds and flu are all signs that the body's immune system is functioning below par. A healthy adult, for example, should suffer no more than two colds a year, so if you do succumb more to every passing infection or suffer from a lacklustre experience of health, you definitely need to start supporting your immune system. The self-defence action plan in the chapters that follow will help you to make positive changes to your diet and lifestyle right now so that you can give yourself a fighting chance of having the most precious gift of all: vibrant health.

7

Eating for immunity

You are probably familiar with the phrase, 'You are what you eat', and nowhere is this more true than with regard to protecting your body's immune defences. Food not only affects the way we look, feel and behave, it alters our skin, blood, organs, bones and muscles and has an impact on our immune system. Food is used to make every part of our immune system, so its strength will depend on the quality of our food. To repeat, when you eat healthily and consistently you give your body the basic building blocks it needs for renewal, repair and defence against illness.

What is a healthy diet?

There's so much advice out there in magazines, books and on the internet that it can be hard to know what exactly a healthy diet is. The basic steps to good nutrition come from a diet that:

- is balanced overall, with foods from all food groups and with lots of delicious fresh fruit, fresh vegetables and fresh whole-grains, and with fat-free or low-fat milk and milk products;
- is low in saturated fat, trans fat and cholesterol and that keeps total fat intake around 20–25 per cent of calories, with most fats coming from sources of polyunsaturated and monounsaturated fatty acids, such as fish, nuts, seeds and vegetable oils;
- includes a variety of grains daily, especially whole-grains, a good source of fibre – ideally around 50 per cent of total calories should be taken in the form of whole foods, including grains along with lashings of fruit and vegetables;
- includes a variety of fruits and vegetables – eat at least five to seven servings of fruits and vegetables per day, since they are an important source of vitamins, minerals, fibre, and phytochemicals, which provide disease-protective effects to the body;
- includes high-quality protein in the form of nuts, seeds, fish, lean meat and whole grains; ideally around 20 per cent of our calories should come from protein;
- has foods prepared with less sodium or salt (aim for no more than about one teaspoon of salt per day);

- includes plenty of fluids, ideally in the form of water (six to eight glasses a day typically recommended) or juices.

Carbohydrates and your immunity

Carbohydrates, when eaten, are broken down into glucose. We need glucose because it is the major fuel for the brain, muscles and immune system. Complex carbohydrates (i.e. unrefined foods such as grains, fruit, vegetables, nuts and seeds) are by far the best way to get your carbohydrates, as they are packed with nutrients and great for your digestion and energy levels. Refined carbohydrates (as found in processed foods such as cakes, sweets, ready meals and white bread) flood the system with sugar as soon as they are eaten, providing a quick flash of energy followed by fatigue. In contrast, unrefined carbohydrates release their sugar slowly so that the blood sugar level stays in the normal range instead of going up and down rapidly. When blood sugar is low we crave sweets and become easily angry or anxious, but if it is steady we can concentrate better and don't have food cravings.

Another benefit of unrefined carbohydrates is that they are high in fibre, which boosts digestion. A clean digestive tract is better for the immune system because if we are constipated there is a build-up of toxins in the body, which the immune system has to deal with.

When it comes to choosing whole-grains try to avoid wheat, since wheat is a common allergy-provoking food. Try barley, oats, rye, rice, corn, buckwheat and millet instead. Choose whole-grain cereals instead of refined ones and eat lots of vegetables, both raw and cooked.

Protein and your immunity

Protein is the basic building block of all living cells. Proteins make up hormones, enzymes, antibodies and immune cells, and adequate protein intake is important for proper immune functioning. Protein deficiency can adversely affect all facets of immune function.

The constituents of protein are amino acids; there are eight that are vital to life and they can be found in lean meat, fish, low-fat dairy produce as well as in beans, lentils, nuts and seeds. Amino acids perform essential functions. Some control memory, sleep, mood, energy levels and how our immune system functions. A poor diet can easily create an amino acid deficiency, and amino acids are essential to make immune cells and antibodies to fight infection. Healthy forms of complete protein (i.e. proteins that contain all eight essential amino acids) include quinoa, tofu, fish, lean chicken and combined pulses and grains.

The amino acids that stimulate the immune system the most are alanine, aspartic acid, cysteine, glycine, lysine, methionine, glutamine and threonine. Those used for detoxification include glycine, methionine, cysteine, glutamine, taurine and tyrosine. If your diet is healthy along the guidelines listed above it will contain enough of these amino acids.

Water and your immunity

Water is the body's single most important nutrient. Almost all of the body's functions, including our immune system, rely on water. It carries nutrients to the cells, carries waste and toxins away from the cells and out of the body, maintains the body's temperature, and provides protection and cushioning for the joints and organs of the body as well as the skin. It also keeps the lining of the mouth hydrated and moist to reduce susceptibility to colds

We lose water constantly through physiological processes such as sweating, elimination and breathing. This water needs to be replenished. The body does not keep a reserve of water as it does with other nutrients. So, our need for water is continuous. Experts recommend that a healthy adult should drink around eight glasses of water per day. Sometimes we need more water because of accelerated loss of water caused by such things as hot weather, excessive sweating or diarrhoea. Don't wait until you feel thirsty to drink water as thirst is a sign of dehydration.

Essential fatty acids and your immunity

Cold, pressed, unrefined nut or seed oils, such as flax seed oil, walnut oil or pumpkin seed oil, contain the essential fatty acids omega-6 linoleic acid and omega-3 alpha-linolenic acid. In the body omega-3 and omega-6 oils are converted into prostaglandins, essential for immune function.

The best seeds and oils for essential fats are flax, linseeds, hemp and pumpkin, hemp, sunflower, safflower, sesame, corn, walnut, soybean and wheat germ. Take the oil daily on salads or in other dishes. The oil loses critical nutrients when heated; so make sure you consume it cold.

Cold-water fish oils from salmon and mackerel are another good source of essential fatty acid. For best results, eat fish and a salad with a dressing of unrefined, cold-pressed sunflower or walnut oils.

The fatty acid of the fish helps ensure the conversion of the oil's linoleic acid to prostaglandins.

What to avoid

The most important food that you need to avoid to boost immunity is sugar.

A high intake of sugar adversely affects the immune system. Sugar impairs the ability of white blood cells (leucocytes) to sweep up and kill bacteria. It also robs the body of key nutrients, such as zinc, that are vital for the immune function. Sugar can also cause or promote fungal infections, tooth decay, skin rashes, mucus production and intestinal candidiasis. It encourages the growth of a number of bacteria and fungi as it provides a great growth medium for these micro-organisms. Sugar affects everyone; but it can have serious consequences for children. Many children who have a high intake of sugar suffer from recurrent infections, asthma and eczema.

The biggest problem with sugar is that it gets absorbed very fast. Sugar rushes through the stomach wall without being digested, stimulating excess secretion of insulin by the pancreas and causing metabolic imbalances. Ironically, the insulin secreted to deal with refined sugar causes your blood sugar level to fall. When it is low you crave sweets and get easily fatigued and irritated. Even worse, all that excess sugar gets stored as saturated fat, which has been linked to an increased risk of obesity, heart disease, diabetes and cancer.

In addition to avoid sugar, the following foods should also be avoided as they place an unnecessary stress on your immune system by depleting it of the nutrients it needs to function efficiently:

- red meat – high in saturated fat, which is linked to an increased risk of heart disease and obesity;
- full-fat dairy products (low-fat dairy products in moderation are all right);
- salt – puts undue stress on the kidneys, which are vital for healthy immune function;
- alcohol (one or two drinks a day is the absolute maximum);
- excessive amounts of caffeine (two or three cups a day of coffee, tea or cola is acceptable, but no more than that);
- refined food, processed food, and food loaded with additives and preservatives;

- fried food and cooking oils and fats found in margarines, biscuits, crisps and pastries.

You should also avoid eating too much and eating late at night, because this puts unnecessary pressure on the digestive system. Ideally you should eat a good breakfast, a mid-morning snack, a healthy lunch, a mid-afternoon snack and a light supper. Eating every 3–4 hours and including a little protein with each meal and snack to slow down the conversion of carbohydrate to sugar will keep your blood sugar levels steady and your energy levels constant.

Drastic dieting to lose weight may also lead to frequent and prolonged illnesses because of the nutritional deficiencies it can cause. If you starve yourself, your body will think it's under siege and pump out stress hormones, which – as you'll see later – is bad news for your immune system.

If you need to lose weight, don't diet. Instead protect your health and your immune system by eating a healthy, nutritious diet, exercising more and watching your portion size. Aim for a slow but steady weight loss of no more than 0.5–1kg (1–2 pounds) a week, as research shows that gradual weight loss is the key to losing weight and keeping it off permanently.

The immune-boosting diet

Putting all this into practice is a great way to support and boost your immune system. If it all seems a bit complicated the general guidelines below should help you get started:

- Eat plenty of unrefined carbohydrates every day, such as brown rice, millet, oats, corn or quinoa as cereal, bread or pasta.
- Avoid any form of sugar and 'white' or processed food. Gradually wean yourself off sugar by replacing it with diluted fruit juice concentrates, barley malt sugar, tea-tree honey and molasses. Better still get that sweet taste naturally from fresh fruits and from herbs and spices such as cinnamon.
- Have at least five servings of fresh vegetables and fruit every day.
- For protein, have two or three servings daily of beans, lentils, quinoa, tofu (soya) or vegetables, or one serving of fish or lean meat. Include grains and lentils in your daily diet to increase the protein content.
- For essential fats, eat a handful of seeds or one tablespoon of cold pressed seed oil every day.

- Avoid fried, hydrogenated fat and excess animal fat.
- Drink about six to eight glasses of water and plenty of diluted fruit juices or herbal teas every day.
- Eat every 3–4 hours to avoid blood sugar highs and lows, and never skip breakfast.
- Cut down on the amount of cooking you do (cooking, especially overcooking, depletes nutrients) and try to eat more raw (preferably organic) foods. The fresher and less processed the food you eat is, the better and the higher the nutrient content is. Raw foods that are rich in immune boosting antioxidants help to build a healthy immune system. When you do cook, grilling, stir-frying and baking are healthier than frying and boiling.
- And finally, enjoy your food! Eat slowly and savour every mouthful. Taking time to sit down and chew your food properly allows your saliva to alkalize your food and stimulates the production of essential digestive enzymes in the gut. This isn't as simple as it sounds – most of us rush our meals and gulp food more than we realize.

Immune-boosting nutrients

Here are the key nutrients that help to build immunity and protect you against disease and allergies. If you're eating a healthy diet you'll already be eating foods packed with these immune-boosting nutrients.

Antioxidants

An antioxidant is a nutrient that protects the cells from oxidative damage. Oxidation occurs when a substance reacts with oxygen – for example when an apple is cut and exposed to air it turns brown. An antioxidant can prevent or diminish this process. Your cells use oxygen all the time for the process of combustion: to burn food for energy production, and to get rid of germs and foreign chemicals such as pesticides. During this process substances called free radicals are formed, which can cause cellular damage and trigger disease.

Free radicals are produced by all kinds of combustion – environmental pollution, tobacco smoking, radiation, fried foods (high levels of heat damage the oil) – but fortunately nature supplies us with rich sources of antioxidant nutrients to disarm the free radicals and come to our rescue.

Your diet needs to be rich in the following antioxidants: vitamin A, beta-carotene, vitamin C, vitamin E, zinc and selenium. Vitamin C is the king of immune-boosting nutrients. It is antibacterial as well as antiviral, and it is a natural antihistamine, which helps with the body's response to allergens. Vitamin A is a powerful antiviral vitamin because its inclusion in cell walls makes the walls stronger and more resistant to attack. It is also important for areas of the body at high risk of infection – the respiratory, urinary and digestive systems – because it is involved in maintaining the mucous membranes of these parts of the body. Vitamin E and selenium are needed for antibody response to infection. Zinc promotes the growth of white blood cells (leucocytes), especially the lymphocytes.

Food sources of antioxidants

- Vitamin A: liver, eggs, cold liver oil, low fat dairy products
- Beta-carotene: pumpkin, melon, carrot, sweet potatoes, apricots, green leafy vegetables
- Vitamin C: broccoli, parsley, kiwi fruit, citrus fruit, berries, peppers, blackcurrants, papaya, mangoes
- Vitamin E: avocados, nuts, seeds, unrefined oils, oatmeal
- Zinc: lean meat, pulses, seeds, nuts, whole-grains
- Selenium: nuts, seeds, whole-grains, seafood

Preparing foods that are rich in natural colours (red, orange, green, yellow, purple and blue) will ensure an adequate supply of antioxidants. Enjoy a rainbow of fruit and vegetables every day for an optimal mix of beneficial antioxidants, including carotenoids, which are found in red, orange and green fruit and vegetables such as carrots, mango, watercress, broccoli and peppers. Carotenoids protect and support immune system cells.

B complex
The B vitamins (vitamins B1, B2, B3, B5, B6, B12 and folic acid) work together and are important for immune health. Vitamins B6 and B3 help essential fats to be converted into prostaglandins. Vitamins B6 and B5 are required for antibody production as well as for making sure that the immune army of white cells (leucocytes) does its job properly. Good food sources include whole-grains, liver, game and wheat germ.

Vitamin D
Vitamin D is essential for healthy bones. The immune system suffers if bones are unhealthy as you cannot move freely and therefore cannot push lymph around the body as effectively. Vitamin D is also

required to deactivate the immune system after an infection, which is important. In the summer months we get plenty of vitamin D from sunlight but in the winter it might be a good idea to make sure you eat foods rich in vitamin D, such as eggs, cottage cheese and oily fish.

Iron

Iron is needed for the production of white blood cells (leucocytes) and antibodies, and without sufficient iron you are more likely to suffer from frequent colds and other infections. Eating vitamin C-rich foods at the same time as iron-rich foods will boost absorption of the iron. Good food sources include eggs, whole-grains, green leafy vegetables, lentils, nuts and seeds.

Calcium

Although best known for its effect on bones and teeth, calcium is also important for efficient functioning of the immune system. Good food sources include low-fat dairy products, fortified soya products, seeds, tinned fish with bones, and dark green vegetables such as broccoli and kale.

Magnesium

Magnesium is required for antibody production, and low magnesium levels increase the risk of allergic reactions. This is because a deficiency of magnesium can cause histamine levels to rise. Good food sources include nuts, seeds, green leafy vegetables, root vegetables, egg yolks, whole-grains and dried fruit.

Immune system superfoods

Avocado

Avocado provides vitamins E and B6, which both contribute to the production of antibodies and also to the responsiveness of specialist white blood cells (leucocytes). This delicious fruit also provides lots of skin-enhancing antioxidants, including vitamin C. Slice some and slip it into salads and sandwiches to top up your nutritional intake.

Blackcurrants and blueberries

Blackcurrants and blueberries are rich in vitamin C and help to strengthen the immune system. You can now buy tinned blackcurrants in juice that isn't sugar-laden. Blueberries are naturally sweet and can be eaten raw or in low fat muffins.

Broccoli

Broccoli is packed with antioxidant power as well as being a rich source of fatigue-beating iron, indoles and chlorophyll, which are powerful anti-cancer compounds.

Chillies

Chillies contain vitamin C and other antioxidants. The heat of chilli is thanks to a phytochemical called capsicain, which, amongst other things, can make your nose run. But this can actually help relieve nasal congestion by thinning down mucus in the sinuses.

Cinnamon

This culinary spice has wonderful antibacterial and antifungal properties. It warms the whole system and acts as a tonic, combating weakness during viral infections. To make a warm toddy fill a mug with hot water and add two teaspoons of tea-tree honey, the juice of a lemon and one-quarter of a cinnamon stick. Allow to steep for 10 minutes, then remove the cinnamon stick and enjoy.

Citrus fruits

All citrus fruits are great providers of vitamin C and other beneficial antioxidants. Low vitamin C levels are linked to reduced immunity. Vitamin C also promotes wound healing and helps to keep the skin healthy, thereby supporting a vital first-line defence against infections.

Fish and shellfish

Fish and shellfish provide zinc and vitamin B6, which are needed for efficient infection-fighting white blood cells (leucocytes). Seafood is also a good source of selenium, which is an antioxidant and aids the effective function of many parts of the immune system.

Garlic

Garlic has been used for centuries as a natural antibiotic, antifungal and antiviral remedy. Its pungent sulphur compounds are thought to be what makes it so beneficial. Garlic also contains antioxidants. Crush it into sauces and stews, roast it alongside meat, and mash it with avocado and lemon juice to make a mean, immune system-friendly guacamole.

Nuts and seeds

Nuts and seeds pack in protein, zinc, B vitamins, vitamin E, selenium, magnesium and essential fats. Pumpkin seeds are an especially good source of zinc (needed for healthy skin, and proper function of the thymus and white blood cells), and Brazil nuts are a particularly good source of selenium. Almonds, hazelnuts and sunflower seeds are best for vitamin E. Flax seeds are great for omega-3, and sunflower seeds for omega-6, protein and B vitamins.

Parsley

Parsley is rich in antioxidant vitamins A and C as well as iron, magnesium and cancer-fighting chlorophyll. It is a must for every healthy fridge, back garden or window box.

Seaweed

A wealth of natural trace minerals, vitamins and amino acids can be found in seaweeds. There are many different types, the most popular being nori. Try adding a little to your soups or mix it with mashed potato.

Shitake mushrooms

Shitake mushrooms are superb immune boosters that possess antibacterial, antiviral and anti-parasitic properties. They are a natural source of interferon, which provides protection against viruses. They are also a good source of germanium, an element that enhances immunity. Shitake mushroom are great in stews, soups and stir-fries.

Spinach

Spinach is rich in carotenoids, which the body converts to vitamin A to help to trigger the immune response. The vitamin C content of spinach keeps skin and mucous membranes healthy, while its B vitamins improve energy and nervous system conditions. Spinach is also rich in zinc, required to promote T cell activity. Spinach risotto is a delicious, warming, immune-boosting dish.

Seeds, pulses, nuts and grains

Sprouted seeds, pulses, nuts and grains are bursting with nutrients and live enzymes that can strengthen your immunity. This is because when you eat sprouted seeds you are eating foods that are still in the process of actually growing, and the nutritional power responsible for this growth is at its most intense. All you need to do is take a handful of seeds, pulses and grains and place them in a bowl. Pick over the seeds and remove any broken ones or dirt. Rinse well and soak overnight in tepid water for 12 hours. Then drain them and put them in a jam jar. Rinse them twice a day in a colander for the next few days until they sprout.

Boost your child's immune system

A child's immune system is not fully developed before the age of 14, making children under this age particularly susceptible to infection and illness. What little immunity they do start life with is passed on from the mother via the placenta (before birth) and then in breast milk. This is known as passive immunity and is fairly short-lived.

A more active and longer-lasting immunity is acquired following exposure to infection, which then stimulates the immune system to respond. This exposure can be to an infection like the common cold, caught from someone else, or through immunization.

Poor diet and, as you'll see later, stress are the immune system's enemies, so to boost your child's immune system you need to make sure he or she eats healthily according to the guidelines given in this chapter; gets good antioxidant support to clear out the free radicals that are a normal by-product of metabolism but which, if left unchecked, can destroy tissues and weaken the immune response; and has plenty of time to chill out. Ideally children should get all their nutrients from their diet but if you are concerned, a good multivitamin and mineral supplement designed for children might be sensible.

Do we need to take supplements?

A healthy diet is the basis of good health and having such a diet is one of the best things you can do to boost immunity. In an ideal world we would all be able to get our nutrients from the food we eat. However, we don't live in an ideal world; we live in a world where the food readily available to us is either nutrient-depleted or loaded with additives and preservatives and other toxins that our bodies don't need. Add to that our increasingly busy lives, in which eating on-the-go has become the norm, and it is easy to see how nutritional deficiencies can build up.

The first step to improving your nutrient status is to include more nutrient-rich foods in your diet. It might also be a good idea to take an all-round, good-quality multivitamin supplement, as research[2,3] has shown that people who take multivitamins tend to have less infections than those who do not. Do bear in mind, though, that a multivitamin should never be a substitute for a healthy diet as the healthiest way to get your nutrients is through the food you eat. Think of your multivitamin as your back up or insurance policy when you might be in danger of nutrient deficiency.

To boost immunity, take a good-quality multivitamin and mineral supplement every day providing at least 10,000 international units of vitamin A, 150mg of vitamin E, 25–50mg of B vitamins, 200–400mg of calcium and magnesium, 50mcg of selenium and 10g of zinc. Depending on your circumstances you might also want to take additional vitamin C and antioxidant complex.

A supplement of coenzyme Q10 (30–90mg a day) may also be beneficial. Coenzyme Q10 is found in every cell of your body and is crucial for the health of cells, tissues and organs. It is an antioxidant enzyme that helps to counter damage to the immune system caused by ageing or illness. Some people have successfully treated gum disease using coenzyme Q10 alone, and it is also a great energy booster. Food sources of coenzyme Q10 include fish, organ meats (such as liver, heart and kidney) and the germ portion of whole-grains.

Note: consult your pharmacist or doctor before taking any nutritional supplements as large doses can be toxic.

Probiotic supplements

The average person has about 400 different types of friendly bacteria, mainly resident in the digestive tract. These bacteria are your first line of defence against unfriendly bacteria and disease-producing viruses. They also make sure we digest our food properly, allowing us to get as many nutrients as possible.

Bacterial balance of the digestive tract is important. Few people realize that the digestive tract is actually the largest immune organ in the body and that healthy bowel bacteria can make a real difference to immune health. Symptoms of disturbed digestive health can include excessive wind, bouts of abdominal bloating, thrush, loose stools, constipation or unexplained tiredness. One of the most common digestive disorders is one you may not even know you have. Dysbiosis is the term used to describe an imbalance of the bacteria in the gut. In the right proportions, these bacteria promote good health and boost immunity; however, when this balance is upset the imbalance can cause conditions like irritable bowel syndrome (IBS) or worse.

In a normal gut, there will be, typically, about 1.5kg (3 pounds) of bacteria but the so-called friendly ones, which help with digestion, are outnumbered by those that can cause problems. At best, the good bacteria make up about a third of the population. At worst, especially if you've taken antibiotics for a while or just eaten a bad diet for years, there may be so few good bacteria they're almost non-existent. Keep beneficial bacteria in good shape by eating lots of fibre from fruit, vegetables and whole-grains such as brown rice and oats. You can also eat live 'bio' yoghurt daily or take a *Bifidobacteria* and *Lactobacillus acidophilus* supplement.

Eating live yoghurt can help repopulate levels of good bacteria (or 'friendly' *Lactobacillus* and *Bifidobacteria*), which act as part of the body's defence system, but the trouble here is that you don't know which strain of bacteria you're eating. With probiotic supplements, you know you're getting the *Bifidobacteria*, which, in the right proportions, can help to lower cholesterol levels, to prevent food poisoning, to digest lactose (which is the sugar in milk) and to make the B vitamins, which protect against heart disease. With a probiotic supplement, you'll know that with every capsule, you're ingesting around 4 billion live bacteria of exactly the right strain. To keep them alive, you keep the supplement in the fridge.

You may also want to take a supplement of fructo-oligosaccharides (FOS). These are sweet-tasting substances derived from plants. They feed the good bacteria, encouraging them to multiply and they act in the body like fibre. They occur naturally in bananas, onions, garlic and artichokes – but you'd have to eat these by the bucketful to get a therapeutic dose, so most people buy them in the form of a powder or syrup.

Extra vitamins for older adults

The elderly get sick more easily than younger adults, take longer to recover and are more likely to develop life-threatening illnesses. In fact, infections are the fourth leading cause of death in the elderly. Although the immune system declines naturally with age, an insufficient diet can make matters worse.

Several surveys have shown that almost one-third of apparently healthy elderly people get too little iron, zinc, beta-carotene, and vitamins B6, C and E. Correcting these deficiencies with supplements has successfully strengthened the immune response. Although heredity may play a role in immune system decline, some researchers now feel that reduced immunity need not inevitably accompany ageing. Indeed, 20–25 per cent of older people maintain immune systems as vigorous as those of younger adults, even into their 70s and 80s.

Ideally, the elderly should build up their immune systems by eating more fruit, vegetables and other nutrient-rich foods. Unfortunately, however, those who have lost a spouse or live alone are often not motivated to prepare healthy meals. Some senior citizens cannot get out to the shops, others have lost their teeth, have other medical problems that require special diets, or are taking medications that leech nutrients.

Although research is not yet conclusive for all these reasons, extra vitamin and mineral supplements may be a good idea for some older people.

What to eat or not eat when you're sick

The old saying about 'starving a fever' is right. In fact, it appears that loss of appetite is the body's way of saying that you should eat less while it battles foreign micro-organisms. As part of this strategy, the body usually withdraws antioxidant nutrients from the bloodstream and stores them in the liver, thymus and bone marrow so that bacteria can't snap them up.

Well-nourished, healthy adults can deal with the nutritional depletion caused by infection. But extra care is needed for children, the elderly and anybody who is sick more for than about 5 days or who loses 5 per cent of bodyweight. A vitamin or mineral supplement or a liquid nutritional supplement taken under a doctor's supervision may be helpful.

When the fever breaks, drink lots of water and other fluids – especially citrus juice – to replace the fluid you have lost. Also, eat grapes, juicy fruits, milk shakes, broth and whole-grain breads. They can help replace the missing nutrients.

'Feeding a cold' is another piece of folklore that turns out to be correct. Hot, spicy foods, such as chilli peppers, horseradish, black and red pepper, garlic, and pepper sauce, may stimulate mucus flow and relieve symptoms of asthma, bronchitis, sinus trouble and colds. However, people with asthma who are taking theophylline should not feed their cold charcoal-broiled meat, broccoli or cabbage. Research has shown that protein, hydrocarbons on charcoal-broiled meat and chemicals found in cruciferous vegetables such as broccoli can speed up liver function and rush some drugs, including theophylline, out of the system before they've done their job.

Science also is finding evidence to support the use of chicken soup as a cold remedy. It seems that chicken soup has anti-inflammatory properties that may help to soothe symptoms of the common cold. It is also comforting and nourishing and provides all-important fluid. Although chicken soup isn't a miracle cure, neither are any of the pharmaceutical remedies.

8

Exercise and skin-brushing techniques

In addition to a healthy diet, regular exercise is another great way to keep your immune system healthy. Just as moderation in all things is the key to a healthy diet the same is true for exercise: too much depresses the immune system, too little is a recipe for a deficient immune system.

How exercise boosts immunity

The health benefits of exercise are clear. Exercise stimulates circulation, improves muscle tone, lifts mood by causing the production of hormone-like chemicals called endorphins, improves cardiac function, and boosts immunity by stimulating the production of a variety of immune cells and enhancing the overall function of the immune system. As little as 30 minutes of walking a day, three to five times a week, is enough to boost both cardiovascular fitness and immunity.

Exercise helps eliminate toxins from the body. First, when we exercise we breathe more deeply, more forcefully and more often. In doing so, we release toxic by-products through the lungs. Second, when we exercise we also perspire. Perspiration is another means of eliminating metabolic waste material from the body. Finally, muscular activity is the only way to move waste material through the lymphatic vessels and, as the lymphatic system contains a vast proportion of our immune defences, it's clearly important that it stays on the move. If we don't sweat, don't breathe heavily and don't move our muscles, these toxins must find another way out. Unfortunately, they usually remain in the body, only to foul the biochemical machinery that makes our immune system operate efficiently. The result: susceptibility to illness.

Researchers[4] at the University of South Carolina and the University of Massachusetts recently studied some 550 adults. Those who regularly exercised at least moderately had about 25 per cent fewer colds during the one-year study than those who seldom or never exercised. Results of at least three small clinical trials tend to confirm this finding. In all three of these trials, women who were told to walk briskly most days for 3 months developed colds only about half as often as those who didn't exercise.

The research shows that during moderate exercise, several positive changes occur in the immune system. Various immune cells circulate through the body more quickly and are better able to kill bacteria and viruses. Once the moderate exercise bout is over, the immune system returns to normal within a few hours.

The preliminary conclusions are that moderate activity, such as a brisk walk, will give your immune system a boost, and that this, in turn, should increase your chances of fighting off cold viruses over the long term.

Getting started

Exercise that increases your heart rate and moves large muscles (such as the muscles in your legs and arms) is what you should aim for. Choose an activity that you enjoy and that you can start slowly and increase gradually as you become used to it. Walking briskly is very popular and does not require special equipment. Other good exercises if you feel more energetic include swimming, cycling and gentle trampoline jumping. You don't necessarily have to join a gym. Other suggestions for activities that don't feel like structured exercise include dancing, gardening and even housework.

How long should I exercise?

In addition to increasing your activity levels during the day (for example, by standing rather than sitting, by getting off the bus a few stops early or by taking the stairs instead of the lift), start by exercising for 5–15 minutes three or more times a week and then gradually and slowly work up to at least 30 minutes four to six times a week. Getting to 30 minutes five times a week may take several weeks or even a few months to achieve, so don't worry if you feel exhausted after your first 10-minute session. Just stick with it and you'll soon find that your fitness levels and your enjoyment increase. If you don't think you can find a spare 30 minutes, try to include several short bouts of activity in a day, say three lots of 10 minutes. Exercising during a lunch break or on your way to do everyday tasks may help you to add physical activity to a busy schedule. Exercising with a friend or a family member can help to make it fun, and having a partner to encourage you can help you to stick at it.

Is there anything I should do before and after I exercise?

You should start an exercise session with a gradual warm-up period. During this time (about 5–10 minutes), you should slowly stretch your muscles first, and then gradually increase your level of activity. For example, begin walking or dancing slowly and then pick up the pace.

After you have finished exercising, cool down for about 5–10 minutes. Again, stretch your muscles and let your heart rate slow down gradually.

How hard do I have to exercise?

The exercise credo of the eighties, 'no pain, no gain', has fortunately given way to a more realistic notion that moderate exercise confers as many health benefits as strenuous exercise. Moderate exercisers have the added benefit of suffering fewer injuries as well. In fact, highly strenuous training can temporarily weaken immune function because high-intensity or prolonged endurance exercise steps up the output of two so-called stress hormones, adrenaline and cortisol, both of which can depress various components of the immune system. Olympic athletes and other highly trained athletes often report that after intense competition and training they are more susceptible to colds.

Exercising too hard and for too long isn't good for your immune system so you need to aim for exercise that is moderate. One way to ensure that you are exercising at the right pace is to see if you can carry on a conversation while you are exercising. You should be slightly out of breath but not panting and unable to speak. So if you find yourself panting, huffing and puffing, stop. You're exercising too hard.

While intensive training is what some prefer, rest assured that something as simple as a daily walk will provide your body with health and immune benefits. If you enjoy sport or other physical pastimes such as walking, dancing or hiking, that will provide a more than adequate way to get the immune-boosting exercise your body needs. The key is, no matter how you get your exercise, to do it regularly and make sure it's fun!

Sample exercise plan for walking, swimming, cycling and jogging

Walking

Walking is great. No expertise or equipment is required, you can do it at any time and it's free! What's more, provided you do it regularly and for long enough, walking can be just as beneficial as any of the more vigorous activities.

How to start

Take a 10-minutes walk, twice a day.

Gradually extend yourself

- Walk every day
- Walk longer
- Walk faster
- Walk and swing your arms at the same time
- Walk up one or two gentle slopes
- Walk up steeper slopes

Ideally

Aim to walk briskly (swinging your arms) for 30 minutes each day. This should include at least one reasonably steep slope. Please note that this may take you several months to achieve, so don't be in a hurry. Remember, exercise is for LIFE!

Swimming

For most people, especially those who are very overweight, swimming is even better than walking.

How to start and then extend yourself

As with walking, start by going to the pool twice a week for a gentle 15-minute swim. Gradually increase the length of your swim and your work rate while in the water. Aim to build up to about 30 minutes a day, or 45 minutes twice a week.

Cycling (or using a cycle machine), trampoline jumping or jogging

Your aim is the same as for walking or swimming. Start with a short easy routine – 10–15 minutes a day – and gradually work up to about 30 minutes a day. Gradually increase your work rate without ever straining yourself.

If you're jogging, please invest in a good pair of running shoes that offer cushioned support, and if you're a woman invest in a good sports bra (for all activities).

How do I avoid injuring myself?

The safest way to keep from injuring yourself during exercise is to avoid trying to do too much too soon. Start with an activity that is fairly easy for you, such as walking. Do it for a few minutes a day or several times a day. Then slowly increase the time and level of activity. For example, increase how fast you walk over several weeks. If you feel tired or sore, ease up somewhat on the level of exercise, or take a day off to rest. Try not to give up entirely even if you don't feel great right away! Talk with your doctor if you have questions or think you have injured yourself seriously.

Remember to begin slowly and gradually build

If you haven't exercised for a while it's really important to find a form of exercise you enjoy and to start slowly and build gradually. Attempting 'too much, too soon' will lead to soreness, fatigue and injuries. Work at your own level, start out slowly and gradually increase the duration and level of difficulty as your body progresses. Getting fit, like healthy eating, is not an overnight proposition, it's a lifestyle commitment. Don't expect immediate dramatic changes in your body shape or health. Although changes are happening internally, most external benefits won't become visible for the first 4–6 weeks. Stay focused on your lifestyle choice and celebrate the internal benefits you're experiencing, such as increased energy, less stress and anxiety, higher self-esteem, and an increased feeling of well-being.

Note: if you have an existing medical condition, see your doctor before embarking on any exercise plan.

Staying motivated

Only one-third of those who begin an exercise programme are still exercising by the end of their first year. The good news is that with some strategizing and planning, you can beat the dropout odds and make a successful transition to a lifestyle that incorporates exercise. Here are some tips to help you stay motivated.

- Find a fitness partner. Studies show that exercise adherence is generally greater if the family or a friend is included in the commitment to exercise. Find a walking partner, play tennis with your spouse or go rollerblading with the children.

- Start an exercise log or journal. This is an excellent way to chart your progress and provide motivation. Nothing beats the feeling of success as you read through your accomplishments. Exercise logs can take many forms: a calendar to record your work-outs, a daily journal to record your feelings and goals, a computerized exercise log, or a log purchased at a bookshop. The key is to select a log or journal that fits your needs and provides the kind of information that is meaningful to you.

- Schedule your work-outs. Exercise must be a priority in order to establish it as a lifestyle practice. Make time for your work-outs and put them on your daily calendar or planner. Don't let others lead you astray. Inform everyone of your exercise time and that you would appreciate their respecting your choice. When approached, invite others to either come along or come back later.

- Make exercise non-negotiable. Think of it as something you do without question, like brushing your teeth or going to work. Taking the lifestyle perspective will help you to make exercise a habit. It takes weeks to form a habit. So keep at it, knowing the more consistent you are in the beginning, the more fixed your new activity will become.

- Be patient with yourself. Some days you will be more motivated or have more time than other days. When possible, do more. When you can't, do less, or do something different. When you can't exercise for a while because of illness, injury or demands on your time, back off without guilt: a brief period of not exercising is not a disaster.

- Set achievable goals. The more easily you accomplish your goals, the more likely you are to sustain them. Set goals that emphasize the process (for example, exercising daily for 1 month) as well as the product (for example, jogging 3 miles in 30 minutes). When you achieve a goal, reward yourself. Decide on a reward ahead of time to spur you on.

- Have fun. Customize your approach to make exercise more enjoyable. For instance, read, watch TV or listen to your favourite music while pedalling a stationary bicycle.

- Affirm your efforts. Your subconscious believes what it hears, without reasoning. Affirm out loud each morning (when no one is listening!) that you are vibrant and looking forward to a chance to exercise. Then, when the opportunity for exercise arises, your mind will encourage you.

- Listen to your body. If you exercise regularly, your body may at times say no. Take the hint. You may be doing too much, and overtraining can dampen enthusiasm, causing you to quit. Shift to a milder form of exercise, or take a break. A respite may inspire you to come back with renewed vigour and determination.
- Dress the part. Wear comfortable clothes appropriate for exercising; they will help you feel like working out. If you exercise at a gym put your exercise wear in a bag and set it beside the door the night before. When it's time to head out the door, all you have to do is grab your bag on the way out.

Warning!

Never overdo exercise! Moderate not intense exercise boosts immunity.

Do's and don'ts

To increase fitness without damaging muscles or the immune system, exercise physiologists suggest several do's and don'ts.

Do's

- Spend at least 30 minutes on moderate physical activity on most, preferably all, days – brisk walking, cycling, swimming, gardening – either continuously or in 10-minute bouts.
- If you run, a good goal is 10–15 miles a week. More than that won't boost longevity or health, and running more than 30 miles a week may be detrimental.
- To maintain muscle mass and bone density, lift weights (light dumbbells will do – or if you haven't got any, use a couple of baked bean cans) two to three times a week. Weights should be heavy enough that you can only lift them eight or 10 times before needing a rest.
- For cardiovascular conditioning, keep your heart rate at 65–90 per cent of maximum for 30 minutes, three to five times a week. To find the right range for your heart rate, subtract your age from the number 220, then multiply the result by 0.6 to get the low end of your target range, and then by 0.8 to get the high end of your target range.
- If you have a serious disease such as HIV infection, chronic fatigue syndrome or cancer, ask your doctor about exercising. Moderate exercise, under supervision, may be beneficial.

- Follow the 'neck-up' rule for exercising with a cold – if symptoms are primarily nasal, exercise as usual.

Don'ts

- Don't exercise if you have symptoms below the neck such as a bad cough or a fever or muscle aches. Muscle aches may be a sign of infection with the Coxsackie virus; exercise can cause this virus to migrate to the heart, with potentially fatal consequences. If you're coughing from bronchitis, exercise may trigger asthma.
- Don't exercise hard for any more than 90 minutes at a time to avoid release of cortisol, a stress hormone and immune suppressant.
- Don't overtrain lest you compromise immunity, especially if you have other stresses like major job problems or divorce.
- Don't lose weight too fast. Losing more than 1kg (2 pounds) a week may compromise T cells. If you exercise and starve yourself, your body may interpret this as stress and pump out cortisol, which is bad news for your immune system.

Boosting immunity if you need or want to train hard

The more you exercise the more your body has to build and repair muscle. If you need or want to train hard, your muscles and bones will definitely need extra antioxidant nutrients as well as calcium and magnesium, so make sure your diet is rich in these nutrients. The most essential amino acid for rebuilding and repairing muscles is glutamine. The best dietary sources of glutamine include poultry, beef, fish, cabbage, beets and dairy products.

Adequate rest after high-intensity exercise is essential. After a marathon, a triathlon or a vigorous bike ride, you need to plan rest days. For up to 72 hours after your event, you should take it easy and participate in mild, low-intensity exercise just to stretch your muscles and alleviate soreness. Gradually build up your training after plenty of rest.

If you have a cold

It's too late – you haven't managed to avoid that cold. Should you rest or exercise to sweat it out?

Animal studies have shown that one or two periods of high-intensity exercise during infection lead to more severe symptoms and an increased risk of spread of infection to other parts of the body, particularly the heart muscle. There are well-documented cases of athletes competing with viral illness who end up with damage to the heart muscle, which may be permanent and, in some cases, fatal.

It is also well established that performance is markedly reduced in the presence of a viral infection. In addition, exercising when sick can lead to 'post-viral fatigue syndrome', in which symptoms persist for months and include weakness, inability to train hard, easy fatigability, frequent infections and depression.

Although research is limited, most experts recommend that if your symptoms are above the neck and you have no fever, moderate exercise is probably safe. Intensive exercise should be postponed until a few days after the symptoms have gone away. However, if there are symptoms or signs of the flu, such as fever, extreme tiredness, muscle aches or swollen lymph nodes, then at least 2 weeks should probably be allowed before you resume ordinary training.

The immune boosting benefits of deep breathing

Research on the link between oxygen deficiency and disease has been active for several decades. Nobel Prize winner Otto Warburg found that oxygen deficiency was often associated with the development of cancer cells. Other studies that have evaluated lung volume and oxygen capacity have noted a parallel between reduced oxygen and disease, with a link between oxygen deficiency and reduced resistance to illness and increased mortality.

Oxygen plays a key role in our immune function. It is the source of the ammunition used by killer and natural killer T cells against viruses and tumours. Your cells must have oxygen to survive moment-to-moment. To thrive, they rely on a complex exchange between the circulatory system and the lymphatic system. Blood flow carries nutrients and ample amounts of oxygen into the capillaries, while a healthy lymphatic system carries away destructive toxins. Proper breathing is the moderator of this exchange.

Many of us breathe too fast for the conditions in which we find ourselves, that is, we actually hyperventilate. This fast, shallow breathing expels carbon dioxide too quickly and takes in too little oxygen. When breathing is slow, deep and full, however, the lungs work more, the diaphragm moves well, and the intercostals muscles, the back muscles and the abdominal muscles work, drawing in extra oxygen to the bloodstream. Increased oxygenation boost circulation and stimulates healthy functioning of cells, glands and muscles.

Exercise is one way to increase the intake of oxygen and to improve its circulation (aerobic exercise after all means exercise 'with oxygen'), but immune-boosting benefits[5] may also be obtained from deep breathing exercises, such as those outlined below.

Pursed-lip breathing

1 Inhale slowly through your nose until your lungs fill up with air.
2 Purse your lips as if you were going to whistle or kiss someone.
3 Breathe out slowly while keeping your lips pursed.
4 Take twice as long to breathe out as you do to breathe in.
5 Do not force your lungs to empty.

Pursed-lip breathing will help you to control your breathing rate and shortness of breath. It helps more air to get into your lungs and reduces the energy required to breathe. It will also help you to feel more in control and make it easier for you to do things.

Holding your breath

1 Breathe in.
2 Try to hold your breath for 3 seconds.
3 Breathe out.

Holding your breath extends the time for your lungs to exchange oxygen for carbon dioxide. This helps your blood to take in more oxygen.

Breathing from your diaphragm

Your diaphragm is a thick, flat muscle just below your rib-cage and above your abdomen (your belly). By using your diaphragm when you breathe in, you help your lungs to expand so that they take in more air.

1 Relax your shoulders.
2 Put one hand on your abdomen.
3 Make your abdomen push out while you breathe in through your nose.
4 Suck in your abdominal muscles.
5 Breathe out using the pursed-lip technique. You should feel your abdomen go down.

6 Repeat three times and rest for 2 minutes.
7 Repeat this exercise many times a day.

Rib-cage breathing

1 Repeat the steps used in diaphragm breathing, but place your hands on your ribs instead of your abdomen, and don't pull in your abdominal muscles.
2 Feel your chest expand and fall back as you breathe.

These methods will make breathing less work, control your breathing when it's hard to breathe, and help more air get to your lungs and the air sacs where oxygen reaches your bloodstream.

Immune-boosting health benefits of qigong, tai chi and yoga

The slow movements and controlled stretching postures of oriental disciplines such as qigong and yoga can improve muscle strength, flexibility, range of motion, balance, breathing and blood circulation and can promote mental focus, clarity and calmness. Many of the health benefits of these disciplines are, however, due to the fact that they combine deep breathing with gentle exercise to relax the nervous system and boost the immune response.

Qigong and tai chi include exercises that are performed in total stillness as meditative breathing exercises. They also involve gradual movement like a dance in slow motion. There are many forms of qigong but the focus is always on breathing. At the same time the mind is encouraged to relax. Preliminary research[6] into qigong has shown powerful immune-boosting effects for patients with arthritis, asthma, cancer, chronic pain, diabetes, stroke and ulcers. Both qigong and tai chi have been found to promote antibody production.

Yoga is often likened to stretching, but because it involves the breath and the mind it is actually much more than this. It also encourages circulation while stimulating optimal function of the internal organs. In addition, the breathing exercises and meditation practices have been found to reduce stress, to lower blood pressure and to slow the ageing process. Recent research[7] has also found benefit for a number of conditions, including asthma and heart disease.

If you find the practice of yoga, qigong or tai chi appealing, the best way to start is to seek out a class or private teacher. If this isn't possible, a video can be helpful for learning some of the basic movements, which can be practised at home.

Lymphatic stimulation

As we've seen, the lymphatic system is the part of the body responsible for cleansing soft tissue found just under the skin. It's a network of tiny vessels throughout the body, which transports toxins, bacteria, viruses and dead cells to lymph nodes. It's the job of the lymph nodes to break down, deactivate and purify these waste products so they are more easily handled by the organs of elimination, such as the liver and kidneys.

A milky white fluid called lymph carries impurities and waste away from the tissues and passes through gland-like structures spaced throughout the lymphatic system that act as filtering valves. The lymph does not circulate as the blood does, so its movement depends largely on the squeezing effect of muscle contractions. That's why exercise is so great for stimulating lymph flow.

When your lymph isn't circulating efficiently you are more likely to succumb to infection and to feel unwell. You're also more likely to have dark circles under your eyes, puffiness and a pale complexion (all signs of a sluggish lymphatic system). Exercise is the most effective way to stimulate the passage of lymph through the nodes, but positive effects can be achieved through massage and body brushing.

Massage

The direct mechanical effect of rhythmically applied manual pressure and movement used in massage can dramatically increase the rate of blood and lymph flow and by so doing encourage the elimination of toxins and boost your immunity.

Many people consider massage a pampering experience, but it has important health benefits. In fact, you get the most benefit when it is part of your regular wellness routine. There are many different types of massage, including Swedish massage, deep-tissue massage, lymphatic drainage, reflexology, shiatsu and Ayurvedic massage. You need to find what works best for you. If you simply haven't got time for a professional massage, you can give yourself a massage, although it's not as relaxing as being massaged by someone else.

How to give yourself a relaxation massage

- Plan to be undisturbed for an hour or longer. Choose a convenient time when you won't be disturbed, such as before sleeping.
- Play some soft music to help you to relax and stop thinking.
- Use lotion or vegetable oil.

71

- Massage the entire body, or just do part if you don't have time to massage everywhere. Massaging your feet can help relax your entire body or help induce sleep. Face and scalp massage can also be very relaxing.
- Do the massage on the floor or in bed. Adjust your position to be able to reach and work on areas without getting tired. The back is hard to reach so just do the best you can. Whatever area you are working with, position yourself in a way that is comfortable for you. For full body massage, you might start with your feet and progress upwards, or start with your head and progress downwards.
- Use easy, non-tiring massage strokes. Strokes include gliding, rubbing, grabbing, pulling and application of pressure. Slow gliding strokes are best for relaxation and calming. Even applying simple pressure on a sore place can help release tight spots.

Dry skin brushing

Dry skin brushing is another way to stimulate your lymphatic system and boost immunity.[8] The skin is the body's largest organ. During every 24-hour period, the body makes new skin. When the skin functions efficiently, it eliminates 1kg (2 pounds) of waste acids daily, so its ability to excrete toxins is of paramount importance. When the skin ceases to function properly, an increased burden is placed on the lymphatic system and other excretory organs. Dry skin brushing removes the top layer of skin, which helps the skin to excrete toxins and other acids in the body.

The technique for dry skin brushing is simple. With a long-handled, firm, natural bristle bath brush, beginning at the soles of the feet and working your way up the legs, torso, back, hands and arms. In a circular motion, and always toward the heart, brush away the dry, top layer of dead skin.

Daily dry skin brushing for 2–4 minutes is easy to fit into your morning grooming regimen. It's a great opportunity to remove dead skin cells, help remove toxins excreted by the skin, and boost your immunity by improving blood and lymphatic circulation.

9

Balancing hygiene

A crucial but often overlooked step in preventing illness is good hygiene. It is important to wash your hands regularly and to keep your living and working environment as clean as possible. Having said this, another school of thought suggests that we may be too clean and that an infusion of dirt and germs is needed to help the immune system build up its defence. So just how important is good hygiene?

Wash your hands, please

Hand washing is a simple habit – one that requires minimal training and no special equipment. Yet it's without doubt one of the best ways to avoid getting sick. This is because throughout the day you accumulate germs on your hands from a variety of sources, such as direct contact with people, contaminated surfaces, foods, even animals and animal waste. If you don't wash your hands frequently enough, you can infect yourself with these germs by touching your eyes, nose or mouth. And you can spread these germs to others by touching them or by touching surfaces that they also touch, such as doorknobs, towels and taps.

Infectious diseases commonly spread through hand-to-hand contact include the common cold, flu and several gastrointestinal disorders, such as infectious diarrhoea. Inadequate hand hygiene also contributes to food-related illnesses, such as salmonella and *E. coli* infection. According to the US Centers for Disease Control and Prevention, as many as 76 million people in the USA contract a food-borne illness each year. Of these, about 5,000 die as a result of their illness. Others experience the annoying symptoms of nausea, vomiting and diarrhoea.

Keep your living and working environment as clean as possible

If you don't keep your living and working environment as clean as possible you can also infect yourself with germs. This does not mean creating a sterile environment, because exposure to germs is part of life, but the risk can be minimized by following the suggestions below.

Kitchen hygiene

Although the kitchen sink harbours 100,000 times more germs than a bathroom or toilet, most people consider the latter to be the most contaminated part of the house.

- Wash your hands thoroughly before touching food. This is even more important after having touched a pet or used the toilet. Use waterproof plasters to cover cuts.
- Make sure that the sink and surrounding areas are cleaned regularly.
- Keep the fridge at a constant temperature of between 0 and 4°C (32–40°F) and clean it, as well as cupboards, as often as possible. Put raw meat in a dish or on a plate.
- Always check that cleaned surfaces such as worktops and fridges are thoroughly dry before putting food down.
- Wash and disinfect the bin and the area around it (in case of spatters). Bins contain high concentrations of bacteria so it is important to empty them every day and to wash them regularly.
- Towels and cloths and sponges used in the kitchen should be changed frequently and always washed carefully. Surveys reveal that while one person in three changes them every day and 57 per cent at least once a week, 21 million Europeans (7 per cent of the population) change kitchen linen only if it is really dirty or when they think of it.

Bathroom hygiene

The warm and damp atmosphere of a bathroom encourages bacterial growth. Soapy water loaded with bodily bacteria collects in thin layers on the surfaces of the shower, the bath and the shower curtain. If the curtain is made of fabric then it may be machine-washable at a low temperature.

Face flannels remain popular, but their almost constant humidity makes them an ideal breeding ground for germs. As a result, they should be changed regularly and preferably be made from thin material that dries quickly.

- Clean and disinfect baths, sinks and toilets regularly.
- Don't forget doors, handles, toilet rims and taps.
- Hang towels up to dry after use.

- Give each family member his or her own towel.
- Air the room regularly to help to disperse steam.

Dust mites

House dust is a significant source of allergens (substances responsible for causing allergic reactions in some people), of which dust mites are the most important. Dust mites are tiny animals, invisible to the naked eye, which live in fabric, wool and feathers. Dust mites love heat and humidity. They eat the tiny bits of skin that humans shed every day. They are often found in items such as pillows, woollen blankets and cuddly toys. Dust mites are found everywhere, even in really clean houses. Reducing their numbers or containing their presence means that allergic reactions become less severe or non-existent. There are several ways of dealing with dust mites, which are often best combined:

- washing at high temperature – above 55°C (131°F);
- using products that kill dust mites (acaricides);
- controlling the development of dust mites by reducing the humidity and heat in a room so that they find it hard to survive and multiply; and
- reducing the areas of fitted carpets in a home.

Hygiene at work

Good hygiene is just as important at work as it is at home, and the same rules apply. Make sure that work surfaces are cleaned regularly, paying particular attention to objects, such as telephones and water coolers, that are used by large numbers of people.

E. coli *infection*

Taking the above precautions in the living and working environment, in particular the kitchen, can have a dramatic impact on your health. Food poisoning hits the headlines when people come down with salmonella poisoning from eating at the local fast-food outlet. However, about 20 per cent of the yearly millions of cases of food-borne illness start in the home, where you have complete control over the cooking and cleaning.

Food-borne infections – illnesses spread through food or beverages – occur when micro-organisms such as bacteria, viruses or parasites enter your gastrointestinal tract, causing nausea, vomiting, abdominal cramps and diarrhoea. In 1982 the bacteria *E. coli* became a household name after dozens of people became sick from eating *E. coli* O157:H7-contaminated hamburgers at a restaurant. Since then, most *E. coli* O157:H7 infections have been traced to eating undercooked ground beef.

Knowing how *E. coli* is spread, what foods may carry the bacteria and how to handle your food safely can help you avoid getting sick. Undercooked, contaminated ground beef isn't the only cause of *E. coli* O157:H7 infections. You can also get sick from consuming contaminated:

- alfalfa sprouts
- lettuce
- dry cured sausage
- salami
- undercooked roast beef
- unpasteurized milk, apple juice and apple cider

Once the harmful types of *E. coli* enter your body, they attach to the cells lining your intestine and begin to multiply. As the bacteria grow in number, they release toxins that damage the lining of your intestine, causing cramping and diarrhoea.

Protect yourself by taking proper food safety precautions. For example, never eat undercooked or uncooked poultry. And always wash any kitchen surfaces that have had uncooked meat on them, not just to protect against flu but also to protect against other things that can make you sick, such as salmonella and *E. coli*. Separate raw meat from cooked or ready-to-eat foods. And don't use the cutting boards, knives, or utensils that are used on uncooked meats on other foods.

Another common source of *E. coli* infection is untreated water. Rain and melting snow can wash *E. coli* into creeks, rivers, streams, lakes and groundwater and infect people, because *E. coli* is present in the diarrhoea stools of an infected person. To prevent infection, avoid possible sources of contamination and make sure you wash your hands.

Proper hand-washing techniques

Good hand-washing techniques include washing your hands with soap and water or using an alcohol-based hand sanitizer. Antimicrobial wipes or towelettes are just as effective as soap and water in cleaning your hands but aren't as good as alcohol-based sanitizers.

Antibacterial soaps have become increasingly popular in recent years. However, these soaps are no more effective at killing germs than are regular soap and water. Using these soaps may even lead to the development of bacteria that are resistant to the products' antimicrobial agents, making it even harder to kill these germs in the future. In general, ordinary soap is fine. The combination of scrubbing your hands with soap and rinsing them with water loosens and removes bacteria from your hands.

Follow these instructions for washing with soap and water:

- Wet your hands with warm, running water and apply liquid or clean bar soap. Lather well.
- Rub your hands vigorously together for at least 15 seconds.
- Scrub all surfaces, including the backs of your hands, your wrists, between your fingers and under your fingernails.
- Rinse well.
- Dry your hands with a clean or disposable towel.
- Use a towel to turn off the tap.

Proper use of an alcohol-based hand sanitizer

Alcohol-based hand sanitizers – which don't require water – are an alternative to hand washing, particularly when soap and water aren't available. Commercially prepared hand sanitizers contain ingredients that help prevent skin dryness. Using these products can result in less skin dryness and irritation than hand washing. Not all hand sanitizers are created equal, though. Some 'waterless' hand sanitizers don't contain alcohol. Use only the alcohol-based products.

To use an alcohol-based hand sanitizer:

- apply about half a teaspoon of the product to the palm of your hand; and
- rub your hands together, covering all surfaces of your hands, until they're dry.

However, if your hands are visibly dirty, wash them with soap and water rather than a sanitizer.

When should you wash your hands?

Although it's impossible to keep your bare hands germ-free, times exist when it's critical to wash your hands to limit the transfer of bacteria, viruses and other microbes. Always wash your hands:

- After using the toilet
- After changing a nappy – wash the nappy-wearer's hands, too
- After touching animals or animal waste
- Before and after preparing food, especially before and immediately after handling raw meat, poultry or fish
- Before eating
- After blowing your nose
- After coughing or sneezing into your hands
- Before and after treating wounds or cuts
- Before and after touching a sick or injured person
- After handling garbage
- Before inserting or removing contact lenses
- When using public toilets, such as those in airports, train stations, bus stations and restaurants.

Children need clean hands, too. You can help your children to avoid getting sick by insisting that they wash their hands properly and frequently. To get them into the habit, teach by example. Wash your hands with your children and supervise their hand washing. Place hand-washing reminders at children's eye level, such as a chart by the bathroom sink for children to mark every time they wash their hands. Tell your children to wash their hands for as long as it takes them to sing their alphabet or 'Happy birthday' twice. This works especially well with younger children, who may rush when washing their hands.

Older children and adolescents can use alcohol-based hand sanitizers. Younger children can use them, too – with an adult's help. Just make sure the sanitizer has completely dried before your child touches anything. This will avoid ingestion of alcohol from hand-to-mouth contact. Store the container safely away after use.

Hand washing is especially important for children who attend day care. Children in day care are at greater risk of gastrointestinal diseases, which can easily spread to family members and others in the community. To protect your child's health, be sure your day-care centre promotes sound hygiene, including frequent hand washing or the use of alcohol-based hand sanitizers. Ask whether the children are required to wash their hands several times a day – not just before meals. And make sure the sink is low enough for children to use, or that it has a stool underneath so that children can reach it. Note, too, whether nappy-changing areas are cleaned after each use and whether eating and nappy-changing areas are well separated.

To sum up, hand washing doesn't take much time or effort, but it offers great rewards for you and your family in terms of preventing illness. Adopting this simple habit today and encouraging those you care about to do the same is a powerful way to help to protect your health.

Hospitals and hand washing

Hand washing is a proven method of keeping bacteria and viruses from spreading and it's fundamental to boosting your immunity. One of the major reasons that hospital hygiene has been criticized so heavily in recent years and that patients have caught infections at hospital – the very place they go to be cured – is poor hand hygiene. Hospital workers are not washing their hands as often as they should.

Infection control has always been one of the main concerns of all health-care workers and organizations but, no matter how technical the recommendations for improvement are, the key to infection control remains basic: frequent hand washing. Hand hygiene sounds so simple, but there are a lot of barriers: time constraints, understaffing, prioritizing patient needs above hand hygiene, inaccessible sinks or unavailability of hygiene products, perception that wearing gloves eliminates the need to wash hands, skin irritation, influence of noncompliant workers, lack of knowledge of proper techniques and lack of recognition of hand hygiene opportunities during patient care.

Hand hygiene is the single most effective way of preventing the transmission of health-care-associated infections. Fortunately, new recommendations and guidelines are in place to encourage and insist on the practice.

The hygiene hypothesis: are we too clean?

The common belief that has driven medicine, as well as public perception and hygiene practices, is that when we get sick it is because of something we ate or inhaled or were exposed to in other ways. The hygiene hypothesis, however, points in a different direction, proposing that in many diseases it is a lack of exposure to the 'bad guys' that causes harm.

Increased hygiene and a lack of exposure to various microorganisms may be affecting the immune systems of many populations – particularly in highly developed countries like the US – to the degree that individuals are losing their bodily ability to fight off certain diseases. That's the essence of the hygiene hypothesis, a fairly new school of thought that argues that rising incidence of asthma, inflammatory bowel disease, multiple sclerosis and perhaps several other autoimmune diseases may be, at least in part, the result of lifestyle and environmental changes that have made us too clean for our own good.

The hygiene hypothesis suggests that it is the more hygienic ones who are more susceptible to autoimmune diseases. The argument is – and we don't yet have a proof of it – that the immune system needs some kind of hardening, some kind of resistance to function optimally.

While the evidence is by no means clear-cut, some studies show that children who lived on farms when they were very young have a reduced incidence of asthma, which has led several researchers to conclude that organisms in cattle dust and manure may be the stimuli that their immune systems needed to fight off asthma. Other research found that ultra-clean children were more likely to suffer from eczema or wheezing than children with less hygienic habits. The more hygienic the child, the more likely he or she was to be affected.

Supporters of the hygiene hypothesis have not proposed that 'playing in the dirt', or making society less hygienic in general, are useful goals in medicine. But they do propose that to keep the immune system working properly you need controlled stimulus or else it doesn't know how to recognize the bad guys.

So, are we too clean? Research[9] is definitely pointing to dirty children being healthier children and growing up to be healthier adults. Dirt, it seems, isn't always dirty, and bacteria isn't always bad. Getting obsessive about cleanliness and sterilization and keeping children ultra clean isn't recommended, but this doesn't mean hygiene isn't important. Once again a balanced approach seems to be the answer. As long as you wash your hands at appropriate times and keep your living and working environment as clean as you can but don't get obsessive about it, you'll be getting the balance about right. Life, after all, is for living, not for cleaning.

Common immunity myths

Although washing your hands at certain times during the day according to the guidelines given above is important, it simply isn't true that totally minimizing your contact with dirt and germs will keep you disease free. In fact as we've seen being too clean may have the opposite effect. Listed below are some other myths and facts about immunity that may also surprise you.

Myth: Over-the-counter cold and flu remedies work well for children

When it comes to treating your child's cold or flu, don't expect to get a lot of help from the chemist. The oldest remedies – plenty of rest and fluids – are still the best. If you do decide to give your child cold and flu medications, do it carefully. These products can cause drowsiness, upset stomach, sleeplessness and other side-effects. Follow the dosing instructions, and stop offering medicines that don't seem to be working. (Note: most paediatricians recommend against over-the-counter cold medicines for babies under 6 months. And you should always check with your doctor before giving your baby or young toddler any medication.) Finally, never give aspirin to a child who has a cold or flu. The combination of aspirin and a viral illness can trigger Reye's syndrome, a rare but dangerous disease.

Myth: Antibiotics can kill the germs that cause colds and the flu

This is one myth that just won't go away. Doctors are asked to write millions of antibiotic prescriptions for colds and flu every year. But no antibiotic – from 'Amoxil' to 'Zithromax' – will help a cold or flu. These drugs do only one thing: kill bacteria. And colds and flu are caused by viruses, a class of germs that aren't anything like bacteria. Unless you have a complication of a cold or flu that might nvolve bacteria – such as an ear infection or sinusitis – taking antibiotics for a cold or flu won't help. Not only are antibiotics useless against cold or flu, they can actually be harmful. They can cause diarrhoea, stomach cramps and other side-effects. And when antibiotics are overused, disease-causing bacteria can gradually build up a resistance to the drugs, making future bacterial infections harder to treat.

Myth: There's really no difference between the flu and a bad cold

It can be hard to tell the difference between a cold and the flu, but it's helpful to be able to distinguish one from the other. For one thing, colds almost always go away without causing trouble, but the flu can lead to complications such as pneumonia. Quickly spotting a case of flu also opens up new possibilities for treatment, such as antiviral drugs that kill the virus that causes the flu and can speed recovery.

Here are some pointers to help you tell a cold from a case of the flu. Colds usually come on slowly. The first sign is often a sore, scratchy throat, followed by a runny nose and sneezing. Colds don't usually cause significant fevers in adults, but infants and young children often reach 39°C (about 102°F). Other common symptoms of a cold include cough, headache and stuffiness.

Flu, in contrast, usually hits like a truck. The symptoms come on quickly and tend to be severe. You will feel very weak, tired and achy, and fever may soar to 39.5°C (about 103°F) or even 40.5°C (about 105°F). Other symptoms include a dry cough, runny nose, chills, sore throat, strong headache and eye pain.

Myth: Children in day care will catch more colds than other children

There's actually some truth behind the stereotype of the runny-nosed day-care child. Children in day care can be more prone to colds when they're younger, because they're exposed to more germs. However, they may be less likely to sniffle through school when they're older. A 2002 study[10] published in the *Archives of Pediatric and Adolescent Medicine* found that children who attended large day-care centres during their pre-school years suffered fewer colds in later years, presumably because they had built up immunity to most common cold viruses.

Myth: Breathing the same air as a sick person is the easiest way to catch a cold

Cold viruses can travel through the air – especially when a sick person coughs or sneezes – but it's not a very efficient way for them to find their next victim. They'd much rather hitch a ride on a person's hand. One of the best ways to catch a cold is to grab something that's coated with the virus, perhaps a telephone, a toy or a friend's hand. (Common cold viruses can live for 3 hours on skin or other surfaces.) Germs that stick to your hand can easily enter your body if you happen to rub your eyes or nose, the favourite entry ways for viruses. That's why hand washing is so crucial.

Myth: You're more likely to catch a cold if you're cold or wet – although this myth may be true

Folklore suggests that chilling the surface of the body – through wet clothes, feet and hair – causes common cold symptoms to develop. But past research has dismissed any relationship between chilling and viral infection as having no scientific basis.

In 2005 researchers from Cardiff University, with the aid of bowls of ice water and people's feet, appear to have shown that this is one myth that may be true and being chilly really can encourage a cold to develop. In the UK, we get more ill in winter than in any other country in Europe and the reason may be that we under-dress. Researchers visiting European cities found that, when the temperature drops, people put on hats, scarves, gloves and anoraks. We don't. We stand around waiting for buses and trains shivering, and that is really bad news. When you shiver, your core temperature has dropped so much that your body believes it is an emergency. The blood gets much thicker, which causes heart attacks and strokes, and the immune system is weakened, so you pick up bugs more easily.

It's important to point out that although exposure to cold and damp weather may hamper the immune function of the respiratory system, if there is no exposure to a virus, then it's virtually impossible to get a cold. However, if you are cold and damp and come into contact with a virus your risk of catching an infection is higher. To give yourself the best chance of keeping healthy when it's cold, wrap up when you go out, remembering to keep hands, head and nose warm and dry.

Myth: You can avoid the flu by staying away from sick people

You won't always know who is infected and spreading the flu virus. That's because adults may be infectious for a day before their symptoms appear until 5 days afterwards. Children can be infectious for 10 days or more. Very young children may 'shed' active virus for several days before illness actually begins. You can even get the flu by touching an object that an infected person has touched.

Myth: Public toilets are the worst offenders

It's virtually impossible to catch diseases from toilet seats. Whatever micro-organisms might lie on the seat's surface very rarely infect or contaminate the skin on your thighs and buttocks. Because toilet seats are not major culprits in spreading disease, paper or plastic seat covers offer little more than peace of mind. It is, however, still important to insist on bathroom cleanliness in dormitories and other public areas. And washing your hands after using the toilet is important: touching your mouth, nose or eyes after using taps and door handles that have been touched by others who are infected could spread things such as colds or intestinal viruses, which can lead to more time on those toilet seats!

Most people believe that public areas like public toilets are havens for the most germs. However, the ugly truth is that there may be more germs residing on your own office desk than on a public toilet seat. Public toilets usually get cleaned and disinfected all the time. But most people don't disinfect the things they use every day in their workplaces – including the desk, the phone and the computer keyboard and mouse.

The average office surface can carry thousands of bacteria just waiting to make you ill, so it might be wise to disinfect now and again, especially if you eat lunch at your desk. Another common hazard is the common petrol pump. Hundreds of people use these each day to fill up their cars so make sure you wash your hands after using one.

Myth: Hugging and kissing are great ways to spread cold and flu germs

Don't worry that a kiss or hug will spread your germs to him (or vice versa). Cold and flu viruses like to enter the body through the nose or eyes, so a hug or a peck on the cheek isn't likely to be dangerous.

Myth: The 'air up there' can make you sick

What about aeroplane travel? Can breathing re-circulated aeroplane air cause you to get sick faster? Today's commercial aeroplanes use high-efficiency particulate air filters (HEPA filters) to remove toxins in the air before re-circulating it back into the cabin – and this filtering process is repeated every few minutes. A study conducted in 2002 found that passengers on planes with re-circulated air had no more colds than passengers on planes ventilated with fresh air.

So why do so many people claim to get sick more often when they fly? Take a look at the hacking cougher sitting next to you. You can't do much about who you sit next to on a plane so your best defence is to wash your hands well and often, drink plenty of fluids and get plenty of sleep on your trip so that your own immunity level is at its best.

Myth: Sneezing is a bad sign

Sneezing is a way that your body gets rid of bad things that are in your nose. These things might be bacteria, other germs or other things altogether. You also sneeze when you smell pepper because your body does not like pepper! Sneezing is actually very good for you and your body because it removes things from your body like bacteria and other germs. It also is good because it keeps the tubes that carry the air from your nose to the lungs healthy. Sneezing makes your nose clear when you have a cold.

What's one of the most common ways to prolong an infection?

If you get sick, throw out your toothbrush right away. You can't catch the same cold or flu virus twice, but the virus can hop from toothbrush to toothbrush, infecting other family members. If it's a bacterial infection, such as strep throat, you can also re-infect yourself with the same germs that got you sick in the first place. In that case, throwing out the toothbrush protects both you and the rest of your family.

10

Positive thinking and the fighting spirit

Research[11] shows that stress can greatly increase your susceptibility to colds and other viral diseases. Stress isn't just a burden on your mind: it can interfere with the normal function of your body's immune system.

Immune cells and nerve cells do interact. For example, when fighting an infection, immune cells are able to stimulate the brain to transmit the impulses that produce fever. Receptors for many of the chemicals released during stress, such as adrenalin and noradrenalin (epinephrine and norepinephrine), have been observed on the surface of lymphocytes found near nerve terminals in the lymph nodes and spleen. This suggests that what goes on in the brain can interact with the immune system to suppress or, conversely, enhance the immune response.

Findings suggest that stress-induced anxiety can inhibit natural killer-cell activity and that stress increases heart rate, blood pressure, glucose levels, free radicals and oxidative damage. All this initiates the 'fight-or-flight' response and places undue strain upon the heart and increases feelings of anxiety and depression. Stress also jacks up your body's production of cortisol and adrenalin, hormones that lower immune response. No wonder you're more likely to come down with a cold or the flu when faced with stressful situations like final exams or relationship problems.

If left unchecked, stress can wreak havoc upon our health. Surprisingly, though, it can also have the opposite effect, according to recent research from Ohio State University, which showed that short-term social stress actually benefited the immune system of mice given a low-dose influenza infection.

What this suggests, therefore, is that there are two kinds of stress: short-term stress and long-term or chronic stress. We all have short-term stress, such as when we get lost while driving or when we miss the bus. Even everyday events, such as planning a meal, organizing a party or making time for ordinary activities, can be stressful. This kind of short-term stress can make us feel temporarily worried or anxious but it isn't necessarily bad for our health. In fact it may even boost our immunity. At other times, however, we face long-term stress for which there seems to be no resolution, such as may occur if we experience racial discrimination, a life-threatening illness, a divorce or financial worries. It is these long-term stresses that appear to have the most damaging effect on immunity.

For example, researchers[12] at Ohio State University compared people caring for a spouse who had Alzheimer's disease with other people free of that draining obligation. More than a year later, three key measures of immune function were significantly lower in the carers than in the others. More important, the carers were sick with colds for twice as many days as the others.

In a more rigorous demonstration, researchers at Carnegie Mellon University in Pittsburgh actually sprayed a cold virus into the nostrils of some 400 volunteers. The chance of coming down with a cold was directly proportional to the volunteers' stress levels; those who reported the most tension were almost twice as likely to catch a cold as those with the least.

We shouldn't try to avoid stress altogether because pressure is a fact of life and a certain amount is needed to keep us stimulated. If, however, stress is long term or we just can't find ways to cope effectively with all the pressures and demands that life places upon us, stress can become dangerous.

Ways to beat stress

Learning how to manage stress effectively can mean the difference between being robust and full of life or becoming susceptible to illness and disease. Here are 20 natural and healthy ways to ease stress and boost your immune system at the same time.

1 Walking and physical activity (dancing, gardening, cycling, swimming)

As we saw in Chapter 8, regular exercise and physical activity strengthen your immune system, cardiovascular system and heart, muscles and bones. They also stimulate the release of 'feel-good' endorphins; improve mental functioning, concentration/attention and cognitive performance; and lower cholesterol, blood pressure, cortisol and other stress hormones. In short, exercise is a great way to release pent-up tension and to ease stress. Three 10-minute work-out sessions during the day are just as effective as one 30-minute work-out, and a lot easier to fit into a busy schedule.

2 Stretching

Stretching reduces mental and physical stress, tension and anxiety, promotes good sleep, lowers blood pressure, boosts circulation and slows down your heart rate. It's a great way to ease stress. Full-body stretching helps your muscles to relax and helps you to breath more deeply. Always remember to hold stretches for a minimum of 10 seconds and concentrate on elongating the muscle slowly and rhythmically. Don't bounce!

Tai chi and yoga are great methods of stretching but you can also do 'DIY' stretching exercises, like those listed below, at home.

Neck roll

- Drop your chin to your chest. Stay in this position and feel the stretch in the back of your neck.
- Roll your head to the right. Stay in this position and feel the stretch on the left side.
- Roll your head to the front again. Now, roll your head to the left. Stay in this position and feel the stretch on the right side.
- Do not roll your head backward! You could crush the vertebrae at the top of your spinal column.

Shoulder roll

- With your arms relaxed at your sides, rotate your right shoulder backwards in a circular motion. Be sure to complete the circle while keeping your arm straight at your side.
- Repeat this four times.
- Repeat the exercise with the left shoulder.
- Rotate both shoulders at the same time.
- Repeat three to five times.

Shoulder reach

- Hold your arms straight in front with palms facing each other.
- Interlace your fingers and rotate your palms so they face away from your body.
- Extend your arms forward until you feel a stretch in your shoulders and arms.
- Stay in this position for a few seconds, then relax.
- Repeat this 10 times.

Wrist roll

- Make a loose fist with your right hand.
- Holding your arm still, slowly rotate your hand in a circular motion at the wrist.
- Repeat this 10 times in each direction.
- Repeat the exercise with your left hand.

Side bend

- Stand with your feet apart and your knees slightly bent.
- Raise your right hand over your head and place your left hand on your left hip.
- Lean to the left, bending slightly at the waist. Stop as soon as you feel a slight stretch in your right side.
- Stay in this position for a few seconds and then slowly return to the standing position.
- Repeat this five to 10 times.
- Repeat the exercise five to 10 times to the right side.

Forward bend

- Stand tall and relaxed, stretching through your whole body, and reach up towards the ceiling with your fingertips.
- Then, letting your self bend at the hips and the knees, slowly bring your hand down towards the floor, as far as is comfortable.
- Straighten up and repeat.

Calf stretching

- Stand facing the wall at arm's length from it.
- Place your hands on the wall for support and stretch your right leg out straight behind you with the ball of your foot on the floor, and your toes pointing towards the wall.
- Gently push your right heel towards the floor, allowing your left leg to bend as necessary.

Lower back

- Sit on the floor with your legs straight in front of you and your knees as near to the floor as is comfortable.
- Place your hands on top of your thighs.
- Slowly and smoothly slide your hand down your legs as far as you can comfortably reach.
- Return to the upright position and repeat. Do not bounce into the movement.

3 Deep-breathing techniques for stress release

Not only is deep breathing great for immunity (see Chapter 8), it's also a great stress release. For the next few moments . . . stop doing . . . just sit. Become aware of your breath. Focus on the subtle ebb and flow as you breathe in, and breathe out, and breathe in, and breathe out, and breathe in, and breathe out ... Focus on slowing your heart rate down by breathing in deeply and slowly, then exhaling slowly and completely. Repeat the inhale/exhale cycle at least five times and you should notice a decrease in your heart rate and anxiety level.

You have just experienced a relaxing, albeit brief, time-out. When practised throughout the day, this breathing exercise can reduce your stress level significantly.

4 Eat to beat stress

Stress can deplete our bodies of nutrients – in particular B vitamins, which are essential for healthy adrenal gland function, and antioxidants, which are essential for immunity. To beat stress it is important to eat a balanced, nutritious diet according to the eating-for-immunity guidelines (see Chapter 7). Good nutrition can improve your ability to handle stress by keeping your immune system strong. Fruit and vegetables are a great source of antioxidants, and wholegrains and legumes are good sources of B vitamins.

5 Cut out the chemicals

Surprisingly, much of the stress you experience daily could be due to what you are putting into your body in the form of chemicals.

Caffeine is a stimulant and if you are stressed it will only increase your anxiety further. It also depletes your body of replenishing nutrients that your immune system needs to stay strong. One or two cups of coffee a day is all right, but any more than that isn't good news. Gradually cutting down to one or two cups a day will help avoid the painful withdrawal headaches, but you will feel the benefits of calmer nerves immediately. Don't forget that there is also caffeine in chocolate and in cola drinks.

Alcohol in small doses may help you to relax. However, in larger amounts it may increase stress as it disrupts sleep and causes hangovers. Large amounts of alcohol over an extended period will start damaging your immune system and your ability to handle stress.

Nicotine in the very short-term may appear to relax your body, but it doesn't. Nicotine's toxic effect raises the heart rate and stresses the body and lungs. Consider stopping smoking! There are a number of stop-smoking aids available on the market today.

Try not to overtax your body by feeding it high dosages of sugar. Make sure you always eat breakfast, followed by a mid-morning snack, lunch, a mid-afternoon snack and a light supper. Eating every three to four hours, and making sure you have a little protein with every meal or snack, will help to keep your blood sugar levels stable and your stress levels down.

Limit exposure to pesticides and mercury. Animal and laboratory research suggests that these substances, especially in high doses or with extended exposure, may degrade immune function. A few observational studies have found that people who often work with mercury or certain pesticides may have weakened immune defences. To reduce exposure to pesticides, thoroughly wash fruit and vegetables under running water; use a soft brush and a diluted solution of dish soap to scrub apples, peppers, tomatoes, and other produce that are coated in pesticide-trapping wax. Consider buying organic produce when it's available and affordable. To minimize exposure to mercury, limit your intake of fish that may be high in the metal, such as king mackerel, shark, swordfish, and, to a lesser extent, fresh-water bass, halibut, and bluefin or canned white tuna.

6 Visualization

Visualization is the technique of using your imagination to create what you want in life. It is based on the principle that the mind and the body are intimately connected. Hence you can use visualization in a positive way to beat stress, boost immunity and relax.

Imagery had been found to be very effective for the treatment of stress. Imagery is at the centre of relaxation techniques designed to release brain chemicals that act as your body's natural brain tranquillizers, lowering blood pressure, heart rate and anxiety levels. By and large, researchers find that these techniques work. Because imagery relaxes the body, doctors specializing in imagery often recommend it for stress-related conditions such as headaches, chronic pain in the neck and back, high blood pressure, spastic colon and cramping from premenstrual syndrome.

Several studies[13] suggest that imagery can also boost your immunity. Researchers at Ohio State University found that people with cancer who used imagery while receiving chemotherapy felt more relaxed, better prepared for their treatment and more positive about care than those who didn't use the technique. Danish researchers found increased natural killer cell activity among 10 college students who imagined that their immune system was becoming very effective. Natural killer cells are an important part of the immune system because they can recognize and destroy virus-infected cells, tumour cells and other invaders.

In another small study, researchers at Pennsylvania State University and at Case Western Reserve University School of Medicine in Cleveland, Ohio found that seven people who suffered from recurrent canker sores in their mouth significantly reduced the frequency of their outbreaks after they began visualizing that the sores were bathed in a soothing coating of white blood cells.

Other studies have shown that imagery can lower blood pressure, slow heart rate and help to treat insomnia, obesity, anxiety, stress and phobias.

One simple visualization for general well-being and stress reduction is first to quieten yourself by taking deep breaths. Then visualize yourself inhaling golden or white light or energy and exhaling grey, stale, old energy. The white or golden light represents new, fresh, rejuvenating energy, while the grey energy represents any stress, unhappiness, worries, anger or other negative emotions you may be holding inside you. This visualization is a great way to release the stress and tension of the day and boost your energy. If you have a specific ailment that you are trying to relieve yourself of, visualize the same white or golden energy surrounding the area of your body that is in need of healing. Focus on that white or golden light or energy healing and energizing that area of your body. Continue focusing this healing energy on the afflicted area of your body for whatever time period feels comfortable to you. Try to repeat this procedure daily or multiple times daily if you feel compelled to do so. As always, do what feels right for you.

7 Listen to Beethoven (or Britney)

Listening to music can ease stress and boost your immunity, but it has to be music you love.[14] Something that calms one person might annoy another. Scientists at McGill University in Montreal found that listening to music that gave people chills stimulated the same 'feel-good' parts of the brain that are activated by food and sex. Even better than listening to music is making it, as studies[15] have shown that people who take part in music-based activities, such as playing in a band or singing in a choir, have greatly enhanced natural killer cell activity afterwards.

8 Sleep

Lack of sleep seems to cause some immune-system components to mistakenly attack the body. That may worsen autoimmune disorders such as rheumatoid arthritis and also cause arterial inflammation, which contributes to heart disease. In addition, insufficient sleep impairs the function of other immune components needed to prevent disease; in one study[16] a single night of partial sleep deprivation slashed the activity level of natural killer cells by about one-third. Lack of sleep may be harmful in other ways, too. It contributes to weight gain and diabetes by disrupting hormone levels, and it diminishes mental and physical performance.

Sleep time is when your body and immune system do most of their repairs and rejuvenation. Most people need 7–8 hours of sleep a night. If you sleep less than that or are often tired during the day, try to change your sleep habits. Effective strategies include establishing a regular sleep and rising time, avoiding naps, blocking out disturbances, reserving your bed only for sleep and sex, and limiting your liquid intake – especially of beverages that contain caffeine or alcohol – for a few hours before bed. If you don't drift off to sleep within about 30 minutes, or if you wake up and can't fall back asleep, get up and do something quiet until you feel drowsy. Getting enough sound sleep has a profound impact on your stress levels, immune function and disease resistance. And when you get into bed turn out the night light. Only when it's really dark does your body produce melatonin, a hormone that helps prevent certain diseases. Not sleeping enough, or being exposed to light during the night, decreases melatonin production and boosts estrogen levels, which can trigger hormonal imbalances. Even a dim source like a bedside clock or a night light may switch melatonin production off, so keep your bedroom as dark as possible.

9 Tea

Drinking three or four cups of tea (but no more than four) throughout the day can help to ease stress and to strengthen your immune system and your body's ability to fight off germs and infections. Both green and black teas contain a beneficial amino acid called L-theanine, which can increase the infection-fighting capacity of gamma-delta T cells. L-theanine also promotes a sense of relaxation, calmness and well-being by influencing the release and concentration of neurotransmitters (like dopamine, serotonin and gamma-aminobutyric acid – GABA) in the brain.[17]

10 Take a warm bath

Relaxing in a warm bath relieves sore muscles and joints, reduces stress and tension, and promotes a good night's sleep. Add some soothing music, soft lighting and scented bubble bath or bath foam to create an inexpensive and convenient spa experience in the privacy of your own home.

11 Massage

According to research,[18] massage can ease stress and increase the number and aggressiveness of natural killer cells and disease-fighting antibodies. Treat yourself to a massage for stress release throughout your entire body. You might also like to try reflexology, which involves pressure to areas of the foot that mirror other parts of the body, for maximum stress release. People who experience reflexology say they feel as though they are walking on clouds for hours after a session.

12 Aromatherapy

Relaxing scents can be a powerful stress relief, which is why aromatherapy is so popular. Some aromas, such as jasmine, lavender, chamomile and sage, are a stress release because they may activate the production of the serotonin in the brain. You can put a few drops of essential oil in a bath or on a tissue. Or add several drops to a bowl of steaming water, then cover your head with a towel, bend over the bowl and breathe deeply for several minutes – remember to keep your eyes closed. You can also buy all sorts of vaporizers or oil burners and they can quickly make a room smell very nice. Most of these use a candle under a bowl – you then put a few drops of oil in water in the bowl.

13 Have fun

There is truth to the saying that laughter is the best medicine. One study[19] found that people who responded to stress by seeing the humour or the bright side in the situation had higher blood levels of immunoglobulin A, a key antibody, than their gloomier counterparts. Laughing reduces stress hormones like adrenalin and cortisol. It also benefits your immune system by increasing the number and activity of natural killer T cells. These cells act as the first line of defence against viral attacks and damaged cells.

Find the humour in things and engage in activities that make you laugh to increase your immune function and disease resistance. While painful emotions like anger and grief can impair health, laughter does the opposite. Laughter enhances immunity, increases circulation, stimulates digestion, lowers blood pressure and reduces muscle tension and stress.

Having fun boosts immunity-enhancing chemicals in the body and produces disease-fighting antibodies – which is exactly what a flu shot does. There are several good studies that show that eating chocolate, making love, stroking a pet, being good to yourself and seeking out pleasurable experiences have a beneficial and measurable physiological and psychological effect. So don't feel guilty about doing the things you love. Your immune system thrives on it.

14 Spend time with friends and loved ones

Your immune system likes it when you spend time with friends and loved ones. In one study, researchers exposed people to a cold virus and then monitored how many contacts those people had with friends, family, co-workers and members of community groups. The more social contacts the people had – and the more diverse the contacts – the less likely they were to catch the cold. Another study[20] found that those who regularly attended church or religious meetings had stronger immunity than those who did not.

You might think that isolation from possible sources of infection is a way of reducing your risk of poor health but the opposite is in fact true. Social interaction is absolutely crucial for boosting immunity because it can ease stress and boost the production of feel-good endorphins.

An added benefit to social interaction is that it encourages emotional expression. Expressing your feelings and giving or getting hugs or other forms of touch can all boost the activity of the natural killer cells that seek out and destroy cancer cells or cells that have been invaded by viruses.[21]

15 Turn down the volume

Noise hurts more than your ears. Any unwanted and intrusive sound can trigger muscle tension, increase the heart rate, constrict blood vessels and cause digestive upsets – the same response your body has to being startled or stressed. Chronic exposure to noise can lead to even longer-lasting changes in blood pressure, cholesterol levels and immune function. Research at Cornell University in Ithaca, New York found that women who work in moderately noisy offices produce more of the stress hormone adrenalin and may be more vulnerable to heart disease than women who work in quiet offices. Even worse are unwelcome sounds you perceive as uncontrollable, such as car alarms, barking dogs and public address systems. Try to take control over the noise in your environment, even if it means wearing earplugs or asking the restaurant owner or gym manager to turn down the music.

16 Meditation

The benefits of meditation are uniquely individual, but research[22] shows that it commonly both boosts immunity and relieves stress. To get you started, here's a brief explanation of how to practise a classic and simple meditation, the mantra.

A mantra is a sound, word or phrase that is repeated to yourself out loud or silently. The purpose of the mantra is to discard your normal thoughts and focus your awareness inward. You can select anything as your mantra from a single word to religious scripture, anything that is meditative for you. For this exercise, we will use a natural mantra 'hamsa', being the natural sound one makes when breathing – 'ham' (*h-ah-m*) on inhalation and 'sa' (*s-ah*) on exhalation.

The hamsa meditation

Sit comfortably, back straight, shoulders relaxed with your arms by your side or resting in your lap. Select a quiet place if possible, but it's not essential.

Close your eyes and breath naturally. Sit for a minute before you begin thinking the mantra to allow your heart and breathing to slow.

Gently focus your attention on your breath and begin thinking the mantra, slowly and rhythmically, matching the mantra with your breath – *h-ah-m* on inhalation and *s-ah* on exhalation. Allow yourself to become absorbed in it.

Let your thoughts and feelings come and go without concern. Don't try to control them in any way, simply note them. When you realize you're not repeating the mantra, re-focus your attention on your breathing and begin thinking the mantra again. Don't try to force yourself to think the mantra to the exclusion of all other thoughts.

Meditate for at least 5 minutes, preferably for 10 minutes. When you're finished, take about a minute to slowly return to normal awareness. Gently open your eyes and slowly move to your feet. Be careful not to get up too quickly after meditating – you may experience some dizziness after a deep state of rest.

You may or may not experience a deep state of relaxation and rest after your first time meditating. As with many relaxation techniques, meditation takes practice to reap all the benefits. Don't get discouraged, just stay with it.

17 Get plenty of fresh air and a little sunshine

Get plenty of fresh air – research[23] shows that natural light promotes relaxation and is great for immunity. Be careful to avoid excessive sun exposure, though. While the body needs some sunlight to produce immune-boosting vitamin D, too much sunshine can suppress the immune system. Overexposed skin is also susceptible to skin cancer. If you expect to spend more than about 20 minutes out in the sun from mid-morning to late afternoon during the warmer months in the North or year-round in the South, wear sun-protective clothing and sunglasses, and put on sunscreen with a sun-protective factor (SPF) of at least 15.

18 Write in a journal

Writing in a journal every day is an immune-boosting stress release for many people.[24] It's a stress release not just to get thoughts and feelings out on paper, but also to be able to see a pattern and meaning in our lives. (Some research has shown that cancer patients with a 'fighting spirit' seem to live longer than those who are despondent.)

If writing isn't your thing, anything that gives you a fighting spirit and a sense of meaning and purpose in life, such as prayer, volunteer work, amateur dramatics or campaigning for a cause, can help to boost immunity.

19 Play bridge or other brainy games

Certain kinds of thinking may boost immunity. University of California, Berkeley, neuroscientist Marian Diamond, PhD, found that playing bridge not only encouraged relaxation but stimulated women's immune systems. Her research is the first to show a connection between the immune system and the part of the brain that handles planning, memory, initiative, judgement and abstract thinking. Any mental activity that gets you fully absorbed, such as playing bridge or chess or even doing a crossword, uses one or a combination of these intellectual functions and might benefit immune activity.

20 Look on the bright side

It seems that those with a half-full attitude to life tend to have a more robust immune system than those with a half-empty approach. Years ago, Mayo Clinic researchers found that people who were optimists in their youth tended to live 12 years longer than pessimists. A recent study by Anna L. Marsland, PhD, RN, a psychologist at the University of Pittsburgh Medical Center, found that people who were negative, moody, nervous and easily stressed had a weaker immune response to a hepatitis vaccination than their more positive peers. Another study[25] asked incoming law-school students to predict their performance and then measured their immune function during mid-term exams. The most optimistic students had a more active immune system at that stressful time than their downbeat counterparts.

The immune system takes many of its cues from our thoughts and feelings, so try to keep your outlook optimistic. In a nutshell, calmness, caring, relaxation, laughter, good relationships, expressing emotions, job satisfaction and music are good for immunity. Stress, anger, depression, grief, pessimism, loneliness, repressing emotions, job dissatisfaction, lack of sleep and loud noise are bad for immunity. Optimism can counteract the negative impact that stress, tension and anxiety has on your immune system and well-being. Often it is how you perceive things that determines if you get overwhelmed, both mentally and physically. Having a positive attitude, finding the good in what life throws your way and looking at the bright side of things enhances your ability to manage stress effectively.

Negativity is a personality trait that's difficult to change, but if wearing rose-colored glasses can improve your immunity, why not try on a pair?

11
Complementary therapies

Looking for something more 'natural' to help to ward off or treat the inevitable winter cold? Chances are you've tried some form of alternative medicine, often referred to as 'complementary' medicine, whether it be herbalism, acupuncture, traditional Chinese medicine, aromatherapy or homoeopathy. The term 'complementary' is preferred by many practitioners because they don't see themselves as a substitute for conventional medicine; rather, they provide something that can be used alongside it.

Many – but not all – complementary treatments are traditional therapies that have been used and developed over hundreds of years but were largely removed from the market early last century, after the discovery of penicillin. Antibiotics provided the most effective treatment ever known for the infectious diseases that were the biggest killers at that time. Only in the past couple of decades have alternative therapies become popular again as people become more aware of the side-effects and dangers of over-medication. Although some studies have been done it is important to point out that most complementary have not yet undergone scientific evaluation.

Your best bet is to consult with a qualified practitioner, rather than buy products off the shelf. To ensure safety with complementary medicine, you should tell your doctor about all the products you are taking. If you are on medication, are pregnant or hoping to be, or have a pre-existing medical condition, always consult your doctor before experimenting with alternative therapies.

In the previous chapters mention has been made of a number of complementary techniques that may be able to boost immunity – for example, yoga, visualization, meditation and massage. This chapter gives information on some other popular complementary therapies with immune-boosting benefits.

Herbal medicine

The use of herbal medicine goes back thousands of years, with the earliest written records dated at 2800bc in China. Herbal medicines can be used to treat a range of illnesses, although they are mainly used for colds and allergies such as hay fever. The following herbs are readily available from food shops and chemists and can also be used to boost immunity and levels of stamina.

Echinacea

Without a doubt, the most popular immune-boosting herb today is echinacea. At last count, more than 300 echinacea products were being sold worldwide. Although this herb is native to North America, most of the research studies have been done in Germany. Echinacea has been shown to be an effective antiviral agent against flu. It contains several kinds of polysaccharides that can fight off infection. Echinacea shouldn't just be taken when you've got an infection, though, as research shows it can boost immunity in healthy people. Echinacea is best taken as capsules of the powdered herb (2000mg a day) or as drops of a concentrated extract.

Cat's claw

Although this herb did not gain wide acceptance in the USA and Europe until the early 1990s, Peruvian Indians have been using the root bark for centuries. Like most immune herbs, cat's claw can be used to treat a wide array of disorders related to the immune system, including rheumatoid arthritis, gastric ulcers, colitis, Crohn's disease, inflammation, allergies, herpes, Candida, the leaky bowel syndrome associated with many food allergies, cancer and AIDS.

In one study, cat's claw improved immunity in people with cancer by increasing the number of disease-fighting immune cells in their blood. It has also been shown to contain other chemicals that reduce inflammation, and it has antioxidant, immune stimulating, anti inflammatory and anti-cancer properties. In 1989, a US patent was issued to Klaus Keplinger, MD, of the Immodel laboratory in Austria, for a product based on cat's claw product to help the immune system. The report that explains how the product works states that compounds in the bark are 'suitable for the unspecified stimulation of the immunologic system'.

Liquorice

Liquorice is another great immunity enhancer, strengthening the very first defence put up by an immune system under siege. A tincture of liquorice root is effective against Candida and several types of bacteria, including the notorious staph infection. According to laboratory studies done in the 1970s and 1980s, a compound in liquorice increases interferon production. Another compound impairs the ability of viruses – including herpes – to survive.

Elderberry

Elderberry, like all berries, is good for immunity because it contains high levels of antioxidants. However, elderberry extract has an extra property: it inhibits the action of enzymes that break down cell walls and enable viruses to take hold. Research in Israel showed significant improvement in symptoms – fever, cough and muscle pain – in flu patients who took elderberry extract, now marketed under the brand name Sambucol.

Mushrooms

Certain kinds of mushrooms have been used in China and Japan for centuries to boost immunity. The two most popular are shitake and astragulus. In 1960, American herb researcher Kenneth Cochran, PhD, of the University of Michigan, launched studies on the properties of shitake mushrooms. He discovered that shitake has a strong antiviral compound called lentinan that stimulates the immune system. In follow-up research conducted in Japan, shitake proved more effective than the powerful prescription drug amantadine hydrochloride in fighting viruses. It was also effective against many types of viral infections. Researchers found that one reason for this is that lentinan apparently boosts immune response.

Astragulus has been shown to increase the numbers and the function of T cells and to protect the immune system from damage.

Both these mushrooms are available as powders with the recommended dose being 500mg three times a day. However shitake mushrooms are now sold in supermarkets and health-food shops and they make a great addition to your immune-boosting diet.

Aloe vera

Aloe vera contains beneficial substances, including vitamins, minerals, amino acids, enzymes, essential fats, plus a most potent immune booster called acemannan, that have been shown to boost immune function by increasing the number and function of T cells.

Other herbs

There are many other herbs and plant extracts that help to boost immunity. Some plant antioxidants known to boost immunity – such as bioflavonoids (found in citrus fruit), quercitin (found in cranberries) and grape extract – are sold separately as immune boosting remedies. Garlic is an excellent immune booster, good against viruses, bacteria and parasites. Italian researchers have found that thyme, lavender, bergamot and lemon may stimulate immunity. After conducting preliminary studies, researchers have added eucalyptus, tea-tree, rosemary, black pepper, cardamom, cinnamon, oregano, parsley, cloves, thyme and ginger to this list. Other herbs that have been historically used to inhibit tumour cells in the laboratory are gotu kola, kelp, Siberian ginseng and dandelion. Depending on the herb, the active ingredient may be the essential oil or some other compound.

If you want to take herbal remedies to boost your immunity you might like to consider the following:

- If you feel run down or think you might be coming down with something, try adding echinacea to your daily routine.
- If a cold or flu has taken over, elderberry extract or elderberry lozenges may help you to fight back.
- A daily dose of aloe vera juice and a clove of garlic every day should help build your immunity.

Traditional Chinese medicine

Traditional Chinese medicine has been refined over 3,500 years, and combines herbal medicine, acupuncture, therapeutic massage, and dietary and exercise therapy. The basic principle underlying traditional Chinese medicine is that illness or disease is caused by an imbalance in the body or in the body's relationship to its environment.

Treatment involves addressing this imbalance as well as relieving the symptoms; and whereas western medicine may look at three people with similar symptoms and attribute to them the one disease, Chinese medicine may look at the same three people and identify a different cause in each.

Chinese medicine practitioners claim their therapy can be used for almost anything – from acne and allergies to pain and premenstrual syndrome. Most practitioners, however, will tell you that Chinese medicine's strength is Western medicine's weakness: conditions such as irritable bowel syndrome, colds and flu, headaches, insomnia, chronic fatigue syndrome, skin diseases, infertility and allergies.

There are over 5,000 herbal medicines listed in the Chinese *Materia Medica*, and about 400 of these are commonly used. Herbs consist primarily of dried plant parts (such as cinnamon twigs, bark, ginger and mandarin peel), although animal extracts are occasionally used. Preparations are created by boiling and draining to form a strong-tasting tea, which can either be drunk or applied externally, depending on the condition.

Acupuncture

Acupuncture is generally used for the treatment of pain. It is based on the theory[26] that the immune system is connected to the nervous system: it is believed that the stimulation of acupoints causes responses in the immune system. Acupuncture involves the use of fine needles, placed at specific points along pathways of 'Qi' – vital energy – in the body. This is based on the concept that blockage of 'Qi' creates pain; acupuncture is used to remove these blockages so that the pain is relieved. It is often recommended for people with muscular and skeletal disorders.

Naturopathy

Naturopathy is based on the idea that the body has the power to heal itself if given clean air and water, the right food and exercise, and a healthy lifestyle. Naturopathic treatments aim to restore the body to its natural state of balance.

The roots of naturopathy go back to the ancient Greek physician Hippocrates, who believed that healthy eating and adequate rest and exercise were essential for health – and that cures should stimulate the body's natural healing ability. In the 19th century, this idea was developed further and two concepts central to modern naturopathy were formulated:

- nature cure – the concept that the body has the power to heal itself; and
- natural hygiene – the concept that the body requires clean air and water, regular exercise and fresh food, in order to be healthy.

Naturopaths believe that the body has a natural state of equilibrium, known as 'homoeostasis', and a 'vital force' that facilitates healing. They also believe that poor diet, a lack of exercise or fresh air or sunlight, too much stress, or too many negative thoughts can disturb this equilibrium and lead to disease. It's also thought that an accumulation of toxins in the body – caused by poor elimination of waste products, the ingestion of chemicals or additives or the inhalation of pollutants – can weaken the immune system and suppress the body's vital force.

Instead of treating symptoms directly, naturopaths aim to strengthen the body's natural defences and internal function so the body can bring itself back to health. Many of the therapies it recommends are designed to boost immunity and in many ways it could be said that boosting immunity is, in fact, the main focus of naturopathy.

Naturopathic therapies include:

- healthy foods, herbal and homoeopathic remedies and detoxification regimes (including fasting, enemas and colonic irrigation), which are used to help to eliminate toxins from the body and to strengthen the immune system;
- hydrotherapy (using hot and cold baths, mineral spas and douches), herbal compresses and dry skin brushing, which are used to stimulate circulation and the lymphatic system;
- breathing exercises and stretches, which are used to improve flexibility and promote relaxation;
- osteopathic manipulation, which is used to correct structural misalignment; and
- massage, which is used to improve circulation and relax the body and mind.

Extensive research has demonstrated the immune-boosting benefits of a good diet, regular exercise, therapeutic massage and other techniques employed by naturopaths.

Homoeopathy

Homoeopathic remedies treat illnesses with a substance that produces, in a healthy person, similar symptoms to those displayed by the person who is ill. The mainstream immunization programme is based on a similar principle, but in homoeopathy the remedy used does not infect the patient with the actual disease or virus; rather, it produces similar symptoms to the disease, for example allium cepia, a remedy created from red onion, is used to treat patients whose symptoms include watery eyes and a runny nose.

Homoeopathy works the opposite way from conventional medicine, in which a minimum dose is required for effect. In homoeopathy, the theory is that the more a remedy is diluted the more potent it becomes, the more specific its effects are and the longer they last. It is believed that homoeopathic remedies are diluted to such a degree that no atom of the original substance is left in the final remedy. How the remedies work is not well understood – hence the scepticism of some doctors. Homoeopaths, however, believe the answer is to be found in the domain of quantum physics – the water and alcohol mixture remember that the substance was once there, and they claim that continued dilution and shaking or 'succussion' can imprint the electromagnetic signal of a substance in the water.

Homoeopathic treatments are individualized: each individual patient has a symptom profile and it is likely that two people with the same condition will be given different medicines. Practitioners look at the whole person not just the condition. They will ask a series of questions about the medical history, moods, likes and dislikes, diet, chronic disorders or traumas of the patient in order to draw a list of symptoms, and they pay special attention to unusual symptoms. The choice of remedies depends more on the patient's individual reaction to illness, mentally and emotionally, than on the signs and symptoms characteristic of the disease. For instance, if a patient has headaches, it is not the headaches that will be treated but the person with the symptoms; depending on where the headache is located or when it occurs, different remedies can be used. The remedy that fits all the symptoms of a person is called 'similimum' for that person.

There are over 2,000 homeopathic remedies made from plants, minerals, metals or animals. Their Latin name indicates the substance they were created from. Preliminary research suggests that many of these remedies have alleged immune-boosting properties.

Aromatherapy

Aromatherapy combines healing massage with oils that have the medicinal properties of plants. Essential oils, extracted from the roots, flowers, fruits, leaves and stalks of plants and certain trees, are absorbed in the body by inhalation and through the skin. The scents released in aromatherapy stimulate the hypothalamus, the area of the brain influencing the body's hormone system. It is thought that mood, metabolism and stress levels can be affected by smell.

Clinical research into essential oils in the treatment of medical conditions is limited. It is not well understood how the oil molecules actually enter the bloodstream, but the psychological effects have been well studied. Some essential oils are believed to be uplifting while others have a relaxing and calming effect. They also have analgesic (anti-pain), anti-inflammatory, antiseptic and anti-bacterial properties.

A range of oils is used in treatment (some are not appropriate in pregnancy, for young children or for certain conditions). Trained aromatherapists use high-quality, natural oils diluted in a 'carrier' oil or blended into a cream. Lower dilutions are used for sensitive skin and in pregnancy. Aromatherapy massage techniques are based on Swedish massage, which aims to relieve tension in the body and to improve circulation as well as stimulating the lymphatic system to assist removal of metabolic wastes from the body. The patient may also be asked to use certain oils under the supervision of the practitioner in inhalations: adding a few drops on a handkerchief or in a bowl of hot water, or by using compresses and baths. Light-bulb, candle-lit or electric diffusers are also popular and relatively safe.

Examples of oils that are thought to boost the immune system include:

- basil;
- black pepper;
- eucalyptus;
- grapefruit;
- lavender;
- lemon;
- niaouli;
- peppermint;
- rosemary;
- tea-tree; and
- thyme.

Hydrotherapy and hydrothermal therapy

Water has important cleansing and supportive properties, and hydrothermal therapy makes use of the additional effects of temperature on the body. Different water temperatures, often alternated, are used to achieve certain effects. For example, hot water dilates blood vessels, increasing blood flow to the skin and muscles. This improves circulation and the immune system. Waste products are effectively removed, while nutrients and oxygen are carried around the body. Cold water, on the other hand, stimulates the blood vessels near the skin's surface to constrict, sending blood away from the skin and towards the internal organs, improving their functioning and reducing inflammation.

There are many different methods of applying hydrotherapy, including:

- immersion baths;
- cold rubbings;
- douches;
- sauna, steam room or Turkish bath
- wraps packs/compresses;
- thalassotherapy;
- high-powered jets; and
- whirlpool baths/

Autogenic therapy

'Autogenic' means generated from within. The therapy is a form of deep relaxation, comparable to meditation, whereby a state of physical and mental rest is induced by autosuggestion (the silent repetition of a sequence of statements – typically, 'I am quiet and relaxed ... my right arm feels comfortable and heavy and relaxed ...', continued around the body).

The theory behind autogenic therapy is that by reminding ourselves of the feeling of true relaxation (when the arteries in our limbs open up, increasing blood flow and resulting in a warmth and heaviness) we can actually bring about that effect. The 'fight-or-flight' response to a perceived threat includes an increased heart rate, adrenalin secretion, decreased gastric movement and dilated pupils. This response is sometimes sustained in modern life for prolonged periods of stress; autogenic therapy is a way of switching off this mechanism, which brings both psychological and physical benefits. Through relaxation, the nervous system can tell the white cells to attack the foreign bodies or stop attacking self-cells.

In the autogenic state, natural self-regulatory systems are able to function well, leading to balance between the left and right brain hemispheres, and supporting the immune system.

The training courses typically consist of eight to 10 weekly sessions, alone or in a group, each lasting 90 minutes. The exercises should then be practised for about 10 minutes, several times a day. Autogenic therapy is practised either sitting in a chair or lying down; once mastered, it may be done in almost any environment.

Autogenic training may not be recommended for those suffering from diabetes, hypoglycaemia or heart conditions; it is also not suitable for some people who have a history of psychiatric problems. Consult your doctor first.

12

Fighting infection naturally

If you do succumb to a cold or flu, don't beat yourself up: most adults get two or three a year and even the fittest, healthiest, happiest and most chilled-out person will succumb now and again. And according to the hygiene hypothesis your immune system actually benefits from a work-out every now and again. In other words, just as muscles need to be flexed if you want to stay fit, you need to get sick once in a while to keep your immune system in peak condition.

You can take a variety of medications or experiment with complementary therapies if you're down with an infection, but with no cure in sight for the cold or the flu, current treatments can at best bring symptom relief or shorten the duration of your symptoms. You could also take the 'DIY' approach with the following tried-and-tested home remedies.

Know which symptoms to treat

Those unpleasant and uncomfortable symptoms are, believe it or not, a part of the natural healing process and evidence that the immune system is battling illness. For instance, a fever is your body's way of trying to kill viruses in a hotter-than-normal environment. Also, a fever's hot environment makes germ-killing proteins in your blood circulate more quickly and effectively. Thus, if you endure a moderate fever for a day or two, you may actually get well faster. Coughing and sneezing is another productive symptom; it clears your breathing passages of thick mucus that can carry germs to your lungs and the rest of your body. Even that stuffy nose is best treated mildly or not at all. A decongestant would restrict flow to the blood vessels in your nose and throat, but often you want the increased blood flow because it warms the infected area and helps secretions to carry germs out of your body.

Blow your nose often and in the right way

It's important to blow your nose regularly when you have a cold rather than sniffling mucus back into your head. But when you blow hard, pressure can move germ-carrying phlegm back into your ear passages, causing earache. The best way to blow your nose is to press a finger over one nostril while you blow gently to clear the other.

Treat stuffy noses with warm salt water

Salt-water rinsing helps break nasal congestion while also removing virus particles and bacteria from your nose. Here's a popular recipe.

Mix one-quarter of a teaspoon of salt and one-quarter of a teaspoon of baking soda in 250ml (8 fluid ounces) of warm water. Use a bulb syringe to squirt water into the nose. Hold one nostril closed by applying light finger pressure while squirting the salt mixture into the other nostril. Let it drain. Repeat two or three times, then treat the other nostril.

Stay warm and rested

Staying warm and rested when you first come down with a cold or the flu helps your body to direct its energy toward the immune battle. This battle taxes the body. So give it a little help by wrapping up warm under a blanket.

Gargle

Gargling can moisten a sore throat and bring temporary relief. Try a teaspoon of salt dissolved in warm water, four times daily. To reduce the tickle in your throat, try an astringent gargle – such as tea that contains tannin – to tighten the membranes, or use a thick, viscous gargle made with honey, which is popular in folk medicine. Seep one tablespoon of raspberry leaves or lemon juice in two cups of hot water and mix with one teaspoon of honey. Let the mixture cool to room temperature before gargling.

Drink hot liquids

Hot liquids relieve nasal congestion, prevent dehydration and soothe the uncomfortably inflamed membranes that line your nose and throat. If you're so congested you can't sleep at night, try a hot toddy, an age-old remedy. Make a cup of hot herbal tea. Add one teaspoon of honey and about 30ml of whisky or bourbon. Limit yourself to one. Too much alcohol inflames those membranes and is counterproductive.

Take a steamy shower

Steamy showers moisturize your nasal passages and relax you. If you're dizzy from the flu, run a steamy shower while you sit on a chair nearby and take a sponge bath.

Use a salve under your nose

A small dab of mentholated salve under your nose can open breathing passages and help to restore the irritated skin at the base of the nose. Menthol, eucalyptus and camphor all have mild numbing ingredients that may help relieve the pain of a nose rubbed raw.

Apply hot or cold packs around your congested sinuses

Either temperature works. You can buy reusable hot or cold packs at a chemist, or you can make your own. Take a damp washer and heat it for 55 seconds in a microwave (test the temperature first to make sure it's right for you). For a home-made cold pack, use a small packet of frozen peas.

Sleep with an extra pillow under your head

Using an extra pillow will help to relieve congested nasal passages. If the angle is too awkward, try placing the pillows between the mattress and the box springs to create a more gradual slope.

Don't fly unless necessary

There's no point adding stress to your already stressed-out upper respiratory system, and that's what the change in air pressure will do. Flying with cold or flu congestion can temporarily damage your eardrums as a result of pressure changes during take-off and landing. If you must fly, use a decongestant and carry a nasal spray with you to use just before take-off and landing. Chewing gum and swallowing frequently can also help to relieve pressure.

Eat infection-fighting foods

Try the immune boosting super-foods listed on Chapter 6 and drink plenty of water and chicken or vegetable soup.

Extra vitamin C

In addition to your multivitamin and mineral you might want to take extra vitamin C. Vitamin C is an incredible antiviral agent and research has shown that vitamin C supplements can ease symptoms of colds and flu. Viruses cannot survive in a bloodstream saturated with vitamin C, so take 1–2g of vitamin C three times a day. Alternatively mix 6g of vitamin C powder in fruit juice diluted with water and drink throughout the day. You may also want to supplement this with another important immune-boosting nutrients, zinc. For sore throats zinc lozenges may also help.

If you think you are feeling better wait a day before reducing your vitamin C supplement to 1g per day. Once you have been well for a few days go back to your normal eating and supplement programme.

Probiotic supplements

Probiotic supplements can be a good alternative to antibiotics because they promote health. The purpose of antibiotic drugs is to destroy pathogenic bacteria but in the process they also destroy beneficial bacteria. A single course of antibiotics can wipe out beneficial bacteria for several months, and overuse over several years can actually make you more vulnerable to viruses and infection. Probiotics, on the other hand, are not a drug to wipe out the enemy but a specific strain of beneficial bacteria that can reinforce the body's natural defences. They can be used to restore health in the digestive tract – for example during a stomach bug – and can also be used all year round to build up beneficial bacteria. Health-food stores stock probiotic supplements. Generally you need to take one or two capsules a day with food. *Lactobacillus salivarius, Acidophilus* or *Bifidus* are good strains for adults.

As a rule make sure you see your doctor if an infection has not responded to natural therapies and has persisted for more than a week. In such cases antibiotics may be necessary, but they should only be used as a last resort if the illness could lead to more serious conditions if left unchecked. If you do need to take antibiotics try to take a course of probiotics for a month afterwards to restore healthy gut bacteria.

Remember, serious conditions, such as sinus infections, bronchitis, meningitis, strep throat and asthma, can masquerade as a cold. If you have severe symptoms, or feel sicker with each passing day, call your doctor.

Be good to yourself

The best way to avoid illness, medicines and antibiotics is to keep your immune system strong so it can fight back more effectively and prevent you from getting sick in the first place. So if you feel run down or have just spent a few hours sitting next to someone with a nasty cough or sneeze, rather than waiting to see if you will get ill take extra care of yourself to prevent the onset of an infection.

If you think about it, boosting immunity is really another way of saying 'be good to yourself'. If you're taking care of yourself, the chances are your immune system will keep you fit and healthy, and if you do catch that unavoidable yearly bug, its effects will not be as strong or out as you might expect.

The best gift you can ever give yourself is a robust immune system so treat yourself by taking the necessary steps. Every change recommended in this book will help you enjoy better health and greater vitality. And as you make these changes never forget that life is meant for living, laughing and loving not for wasting time being sick.

The 10 golden immune-boosting rules

1 Immunization. Vaccines for yourself and your children are safe and effective, and they're the best defence against many infectious diseases.

2 Good hygiene. Wash your hands often, especially after using the toilet and when preparing food. Clean and disinfect the 'hot zones' in your home – the kitchen and bathroom – on a regular basis.

3 Make sure there is plenty of colour on your plate. Eat a healthy balanced diet with plenty of variety and lashings of colourful vegetables and fruit.

4 Take a multivitamin and mineral supplement. Even if you are generally healthy and eat well, taking a supplement may act as an insurance policy against any nutritional shortfalls.

5 Get moving for 30 minutes a day. If you can't manage 30 minutes every day, do what you can – every little helps.

6 Make time for rest and relaxation. Get your 8 hours of sleep and find ways to manage stress.

7 Listen to your body. Your body signals offer important information about potential threats to your health: start paying attention to your body.

8 Use your common sense. Steer clear of behaviour that puts you at greater risk. For example, don't handle an animal that looks ill or appears to have an infection. Avoid sharing a drinking glass or utensils with someone who's sick. Take extra good care of yourself if you feel run down. Wrap up warm when it's cold outside.

9 Keep health risks in perspective. Despite the risks that infectious diseases can pose, try not to panic and keep a sense of perspective. Catching an infectious disease may not be the biggest threat to your health. If you're a smoker or you're overweight, your risk of health complications probably outweighs your risk of an infectious disease.

10 Be good to yourself. Have fun, spend time with friends and loved ones, look on the bright side and, most important of all, enjoy your life.

Useful addresses

Immune system dysfunctions

United Kingdom

Allergy UK (formerly the British Allergy Foundation)
3 White Oak Square
London Road
Swanley
Kent BR8 7AG
Tel.: 01322 619898 (helpline)
Website: www.allergyuk.org
Email: info@allergyuk.org

Primary Immunodeficiency Association
Alliance House
12 Caxton Street
London SW1H 0QS
Tel.: 020 7976 7640
Website: www.pia.org.uk
Email: info@pia.org.uk

United States of America

American Autoimmune Related Diseases Association (AARDA)
National Office
22100 Gratiot Avenue
Eastpointe
MI 48021
Tel.: (001) 586776 3900
Website: www.aarda.org/

Immune Deficiency Foundation
40 W. Chesapeake Avenue
Suite 308
Towson
MD 21204
Website: www.primaryimmune.org/

National Institute of Allergy and Infectious Diseases (NIAID)
NIAID Office of Communications and Public Liaison
6610 Rockledge Drive MSC 6612
Bethesda
MD 20892-6612
Website: www.niaid.nih.gov/publications/autoimmune.htm

Complementary therapies

Association of Reflexologists
27 Old Gloucester Street
London WC1N 3XX
Tel.: 0870 567 3320
Website: www.aor.org.uk
Email: info@aor.org.uk

British Association of Nutritional Therapists
27 Old Gloucester Street
London WC1N 3XX
Tel.: 08706 061284
Website: www.bant.org.uk

British Autogenic Society
Royal London Homoeopathic Hospital
Great Ormond Street
London WC1N 3HR
Tel.: 020 7391 8908
Website: www.autogenic-therapy.org.uk
Email: admin@autogenic-therapy.org.uk

The British Institute of Homeopathy
Endeavour House
80 High Street
Egham
Surrey TW20 9HE
Tel.: 01784 473800
Website: www.britinsthom.com
Email: info@britinsthom.com

The British Medical Acupuncture Society (BMAS)
BMAS House
3 Winnington Court
Northwich
Cheshire CW8 1AQ
Tel.: 01606 786752
Website: www.medical-acupuncture.co.uk
Email: admin@medical-acupuncture.org.uk

The British Wheel of Yoga
25 Jermyn Street
Sleaford
Lincs NG34 7RU
Tel.: 01529 306851
Website: www.bwy.org.uk
Email: office@bwy.org.uk

General Council and Register of Naturopaths
Goswell House
2 Goswell Road
Street
Somerset BA16 0JG
Tel.: 08707 456984
Website: www.naturopathy.org.uk

The Hydrotherapy Association
David Butler
PO Box 30
Guildford
Surrey GU3 2JS
Tel.: 01483 813181
Website: www.guide-information.org.uk
Then follow links (provides hydrotherapy equipment)

Institute of Optimum Nutrition (ION)
Avalon House
72 Lower Mortlake Road
Richmond
Surrey TW9 2JY

International Federation of Professional Aromatherapists (IFPA)
82 Ashby Road
Hinckley
Leicestershire LE10 1SN
Tel.: 01455 637987
Website: www.ifparoma.org
Email: admin@ifparoma.org

London College of Massage
Training Venue D2-Diorama
3–7 Euston Centre
London NW1 3JG
Tel.: 020 3259 0000
Website: www.massagelondon.com

National Institute of Medical Herbalists
Elm House
54 Mary Arches Street
Exeter
Devon EX4 3BA
Tel.: 01392 426022
Website: www.nimh.org.uk
Email: nimh@ukexeter.freeserve.co.uk

Register of Chinese Herbal Medicine
Office 5, Ferndale Business Centre
1 Exeter Street
Norwich
Norfolk NR2 4QB
Tel.: 01603 667557
Website: www.rchm.co.uk
Email: herbmed@rchm.co.uk

Further reading

Avlicino, A. *Beat the flu: how to stay healthy through the coming bird flu pandemic.* Fusion Press, 2006.

Burney, L. *Boost your child's immune system.* Piatkus, 2003.

Haigh, C. *The top 100 immunity boosters.* Duncan Baird, 2005.

Hartvig, K. *Eat for immunity.* Duncan Baird, 2002.

Holford, P. *Boost your immune system.* Piatkus, 2004.

Mazo, E. *The immune advantage.* Rodale, 2002.

Saputo, L. *Boosting immunity: creating wellness naturally.* New World, 2002.

Sompayrac, L. *How the immune system works.* Blackwell, 2003.

Williams, J. *Viral immunity: a ten step plan to enhance your immunity against viral diseases using natural medicines.* Hampton Roads, 2002.

References

1. Chandra, R. K., *European Journal of Clinical Nutrition*, suppl. 3, August 2002, pp. S73–6.
2. Graat, J. M. and colleagues, *JAMA: the Journal of the American Medical Association*, vol. 288, 14 August 2002, pp. 715–21.
3. Chavance, M. and colleagues, *International Journal for Vitamin and Nutrition Research*, vol. 63, 1993, pp. 11–16.
4. Matthews, C. E. and colleagues, *Medicine and Science in Sports and Exercise*, vol. 34, August 2002, pp. 1242–8.
5. West, E. and colleagues, *Chest*, vol. 128, November 2005, pp. 3482–8.
6. Lee, M. and colleagues, *European Journal of Cancer Care (England)*, vol. 14, December 2005, pp. 457–62.
7. Khalsa, S. and colleagues, *Indian Journal of Physiology and Pharmacology*, vol. 48, July 2004, pp. 269–85.
8. Iwama, H. and colleagues, *Medical Science Monitor: International Medical Journal of Experimental and Clinical Research*, vol. 8, September 2002, CR611–15.
9. Elston, D. and colleagues, *Journal of the American Academy of Dermatology*, vol. 54, January 2006, pp. 172–9.
10. Ball, T. M. and colleagues, *Archives of Pediatrics and Adolescent Medicine*, vol. 156, February 2002, pp. 121–6.
11. Cohen, S. and colleagues, *The New England Journal of Medicine*, vol. 325, 29 August 1991, pp. 606–12.
12. Kiecolt-Glaser, J.K. and colleagues, *Psychosomatic Medicine*, vol. 53, July–August 1991, pp. 345–62.
13. Gruzelier, J.H., *Stress*, vol. 5, June 2002, pp. 147–63.
14. Nillson, U. and colleagues, *European Journal of Anaesthesiology*, vol. 22, February 2005, pp. 96–102.
15. Kruetz, G. and colleagues, *Journal of Behavioral Medicine*, vol. 27, December 2004, pp. 623–35.
16. Irwin, M. and colleagues, *Psychosomatic Medicine*, vol. 56, November–December 1994, pp. 493–8.
17. Hintikka J. and colleagues, *European Journal of Epidemiology*, vol. 20, 2005, pp. 359–63.
18. Goodfellow L. and colleagues, *Nursing Research*, vol. 52, September–October 2003, pp. 318–28.
19. Segerstrom, S.C. and colleagues, *Journal of Personality and*

Social Psychology, vol. 74, June 1998, pp. 1646–55.
20. Koenig, H.G. and colleagues, *International Journal of Psychiatry in Medicine*, vol. 27, 1997, pp. 233–50.
21. Ester, T. and colleagues, *Psychosomatic Medicine*, vol. 52, July–August 1990, pp. 397–410.
22. Solberg, E.E. and colleagues, *British Journal of Sports Medicine*, vol. 29, December 1995, pp. 255–7.
23. Roberts, J.E., *Annals of the New York Academy of Sciences*, vol. 917, 2000 pp. 435–45.
24. Strauman T. and colleagues, *Brain Behavior and Immunity*, vol. 18, November 2004, pp. 544–54.
25. Martin, R.A., Dobbin, J.P., *International Journal of Psychiatry in Medicine*, vol. 18, 1988, pp. 93–105.
26. Mori H. and colleagues, *Neuroscience Letters*, vol. 320, March 2002, pp. 21–4.

Index